LIMITLESS
STRENGTH

MARK SHERWOOD, ND

LIMITLESS STRENGTH

*Wellness Nuggets That May
Forever Change Your Life*

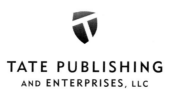

TATE PUBLISHING
AND ENTERPRISES, LLC

Limitless Strength
Copyright © 2015 by Mark Sherwood, ND. All rights reserved.

No part of this publication may be reproduced, stored in a retrieval system or transmitted in any way by any means, electronic, mechanical, photocopy, recording or otherwise without the prior permission of the author except as provided by USA copyright law.

The opinions expressed by the author are not necessarily those of Tate Publishing, LLC.

Published by Tate Publishing & Enterprises, LLC
127 E. Trade Center Terrace | Mustang, Oklahoma 73064 USA
1.888.361.9473 | www.tatepublishing.com

Tate Publishing is committed to excellence in the publishing industry. The company reflects the philosophy established by the founders, based on Psalm 68:11,
"The Lord gave the word and great was the company of those who published it."

Book design copyright © 2015 by Tate Publishing, LLC. All rights reserved.
Cover design by Nikolai Purpura
Interior design by Mary Jean Archival

Published in the United States of America

ISBN: 978-1-68118-580-4
1. Health & Fitness / Healthy Living
2. Body, Mind & Spirit / General
15.04.17

Contents

Foreword 11
Introduction: Totality of Wellness.................................. 15
Practice Makes Perfect.. 17
A Solid First Step 19

Part 1: Physical Wellness

Activity /Exercise 25

1440 minutes—That is ALL You Get 25
The Power of 10... 27
Can Exercising Increase Your Life Expectancy? 29
Physical Activity—a necessary and available resource....... 31
From Contemplation to Action 33
From Inactivity To Exercise 34
Workout 101—Cover All the Bases................................. 37
Balanced Training.. 38
Try This for Increased Arm Size 40

Heavy Weight Training 42
Progressive Resistance—A Must for Growth (Part 1) 43
Progressive Resistance—A Must for Growth (Part 2) 46
Are You Doing Aerobic Activity or Just Kidding
   Yourself?.. 49
Exercise Maintenance—Does it really exist?..................... 52
Training While Injured... 55
The Most Insane Workout Ever—Guaranteed Results 56

Nutritional 59

Time—Want More? 59
Are You In "Wellness" Debt? 61
NOW is the Time for Wellness 63
Solid First Step-Revisited.. 64
Help, I NEED to Lose a Few Pounds 66
Get Rid of the Scales.. 70
You are NOT Meant to Be Fat.. 71
Foundational Eating—Removing the Guesswork............. 73
The 14-Day Meal Plan: How to Effectively Give Up
   Old Eating Habits.. 74
The True VALUE in a Meal 76
Quality Protein—Where Art Thou? 79
Strategies for Reducing Saturated Fats 81
Strategies for Reducing Sugars 82
Taming the Insulin Animal 82

The Great Grain Giveaway 85
Alcohol–What's the harm in a few drinks? 87
Detoxification—a Necessity for Optimum Wellness......... 91
Holiday Excuses 95

Extra Physical Wellness Nuggets 99

Mediocrity is Not Acceptable—Men, Where are You?..... 99
Microwave Mentality.. 102
Misbehavior Justification 105
New Breakthrough 107
New Breakthrough Part Two: Scams, Shams, and
    Quackery... 110
Where to Eat Out and What to Order!........................... 112
What Everybody Ought to Know About Overeating..... 115
Is Cardiovascular Disease (CVD) Preventable? 117

Part 2: Emotional Wellness

Always fun? 125
7 Lessons I Learned that Lead to Complete Freedom..... 126
Generational Wellness 128
How Do You Find Peace in the Midst of Chaos?........... 131
Hyper-vigilance 133
Slow Down and Get Real.. 138
Managing Personal Risk 139

The Exercise—Sanity Connection 141
We DON'T Have to Accept Failure or Mediocrity 142
Don't Miss the Moments 144

Extra Emotional Wellness Nuggets 147

The Daily One-Minute Exercise That Will Change
     Your Life 147
Diaphragmatic Breathing 148

Part 3: Intellectual Wellness

Are You Aiming at the Right Target? 153
Commitment Phobia 155
Consequences—Fact or Fiction? 157
Do You Have a Plan? 159
New Year's STOPS 161
7 Ways to Avoid Surgery—Saving You Boatloads
     of Cash 162
Talk it—Walk it—Live it 166
Re-evaluating Value 168

Extra Intellectual Wellness Nuggets 171

Pre-habilitate Your life 171
Pre-habilitate Your Family 174
Pre-habilitate Your Employment 177

Pre-habilitate Your Business 180
Pre-habilitate Your Church or Ministry.......................... 183

Part 4: Spiritual Wellness

Things Have NOT Been Easy 189
A New Kind of Detoxification.. 192
The Sacrificial Cost of Freedom...................................... 194
Those Eyes.. 196
7 Ways Parents Mislead Their Children without
     Even Knowing It.. 197
Reinventing Integrity... 200
The Art of Uncommon Courtesy 204
Who Else Wants More Time?.. 206
Heroes Wanted.. 209
3 Keys That Will Lead You to Greatness 211
Life without Impossibility 213

Extra Spiritual Wellness Nuggets.................................. 217

How Do We Understand Evil?.. 217
Is Our Faith a Private Matter?... 219
Pastors and the Big Squeeze 221
Physical Stewardship 225

Foreword

"The public has an insatiable appetite for books and products that have to do with health and wellness. The market responds to that quench with thousands of items coming out every year, and much of what the public is given are untruths, schemes and false promises so the search continues ad nauseam. That was until Dr. Mark Sherwood wrote *Limitless Strength*. For anyone wanting true health, longevity and a life changed forever, the search is now over. Whether your wellness efforts include physical, emotional, intellectual or spiritual, you have found what you need. Take it from someone who has spent half a lifetime searching for the answer. Your answer is here and it is time to really live the rest of your life."

Major Travis Yates, Tulsa Police Department Law Officer Magazine International Trainer of the Year.

"Have you ever considered the cost of Ill health? It seems silly to think about. It does make perfect sense when you come to know that 85 % of all long term chronic conditions are lifestyle related. It's like having the perfect car and letting it rust simply because you did not know you need to change the oil, keep up the maintenance and wax the finish in order to maintain it at its optimal performance, and having it fail you at a minimal 50,000 miles when it should run a good 200,000. As you read about the simple things you may know, things you have forgotten and or things you need to put into practice your life will transform.

Within these pages you will find gems to putting the odds in your favor to finding
Limitless Strength:
Discovering the 4E (element) approach to total wellness has transformed my approach to medical practice. It has changed the lens through which I see. Limitless strength put dimension on the overall picture when a patient approaches me with disease. Disease is dimensional. If all four elements are not healthy and whole, wellbeing is not achieved in totality. These guidelines gave me a tool box to guide not only my personal journey but the journey of my patients towards the complete picture of health.

Discover the rewards and joy that come through learning of the 4 elements and how they prosper your sense of completeness. Unfold the strongholds that steal your wellbeing. It takes discipline and an attitude of interest for your own outcome. Its humbling to discover how simple it is to maintain health if we take the important steps to do so. Are you ready to step up to the plate and live a life of "Healing" and "Health" today?

Dr. Michele L Neil-Sherwood is the founder and CEO of the Functional Medical Institute in Tulsa, OK, a medical clinic dedicated to individual health interests and medical needs. She received her Doctor of Osteopathic Medicine degree from the Oklahoma State University College of Osteopathic Medicine. She is a board-certified internist and completed her internal medicine residency at OSU Medical Center. She is also board certified in sports medicine and obtained a sports medicine fellowship through the University of Tulsa. Dr. Neil served on the advisory board at Southcrest Medical Hospital. She is the recipient of the Janet M. Glascow Memorial Achievement Citation; Academic Excellence Award; Phi Kappa Phi Honor Society Top Graduate; The Excellence in Osteopathic Manipulative Medicine Award; and the Internal Medicine Department Award. Dr. Neil has an extensive background in fitness and understands the importance of nutrition/supplementation, exercise prescription, rest, stress management and hormone balance."

Introduction:
Totality of Wellness

Live4E

What exactly is wellness? By definition, it simply means "the absence of illness." To further define and alleviate misconceptions, let me also say that being physically fit does not equate to being well. Additionally, being overweight does not equate to being unfit nor does being slim equate to being healthy. Most people find great confusion in the aforementioned areas. To clarify, let me begin by outlining the 4 parts of wellness. This is what I call the 4E life philosophy.

1. Spiritual. This does NOT mean religious. It simply means that your 'inner self' or 'essence of who you are as a person' needs attention and needs to be 'well.' This requires daily time of inner reflection. This can be accomplished by prayer, meditation, or practicing mindfulness.

2. Intellectual. We need to stimulate the mind. A mind that is not exercised and stimulated can become stagnant. Our minds need the challenge of discovering and learning new information. The mind, not exercised, will become weak. We must have sound and 'well' minds.
3. Emotional. Emotional health is extremely important. Emotions that are out of control can lead you places in which you never wanted to go. Uncontrolled emotion can hinder relationships, jobs, and tasks.
4. Physical. Physical health is NOT an option. It is about the sustainability of life. The components of physical health are what we put IN our bodies and what we do WITH our bodies. Simply put, we must be responsible with nutrition and activity.

The 4 parts of wellness are often treated as separate. In reality they are intertwined and feed into each other. An example of this: When we are active, we feel better (emotionally). When we feel better, we can learn new information more effectively (intellectually). When we learn new information, that information can spur new exploration and revelation into our inner self (spiritually).

As you can see, wellness is really found in giving daily attention to each part of who we are: spiritual, intellectual, emotional, and physical. This is part of the formula for discovering true peace.

In the following pages, you will find bite-size chapters that are easy to digest. The chapters are divided into the 4 areas previously mentioned. There are nuggets of knowledge in each section for everybody. These gems are designed to inspire, educate and motivate you to achieve new levels of the NEW YOU.

This book is about concepts. These concepts represent "pieces" of wellness. It is my desire for you that as these "pieces" are grasped and learned, you will find yourself putting it all together. In the end, you will see these "pieces" form together much like a puzzle. The resulting picture will represent PEACE in your life.

You were designed for greatness. Let's begin anew each day and live the "4E" wellness life together.

Practice Makes Perfect

We have all heard the cliché 'practice makes perfect.' Recently, a colleague added a new twist by saying, "practice not only makes perfect but also permanent." I immediately thought of how that applies to the formation of habits. We can practice both good and bad habits until we become 'perfect' at them and they become a 'permanent' fixture in our daily life.

As we apply this to two primary areas of wellness (activity/ exercise and nutrition), we immediately get a sense of how we can become habitually perfect at making permanent choices that promote either improvement or decline in our wellness.

We must begin practicing good habits in our activity/exercise and nutrition. Let me list some simple principles to live by for each.

I will begin with activity/exercise:

1. Don't begin too fast. Take it one day at a time maybe beginning with as little as 10 minutes of dedicated activity/exercise.
2. Dedicate the activity/exercise at a time that fits your current schedule. Minimize causing a major disruption even if your current habits are less than desirable.
3. Journal your total activity/exercise during the week. If you miss a day, let it go and begin again tomorrow. Don't beat yourself up. During the following week, try to best your previous total activity/exercise time by a few minutes (even 5 minutes).

Principles of nutritional choices:

1. Begin by minimizing between-meal snacks that are high in sugar. This can be done by placing a healthy meal replacement bar or a small plastic bag of carrots, nuts, celery, or apples in your bag, purse, or desk.
2. Try to add at least two vegetables a day to your current nutritional schedule. Don't worry about major changes yet, just ADD the vegetables.
3. Realize that food content is not what it used to be. It does not contain the nutrition it once did.

Supplementation is likely necessary. Eat as many natural and REAL (unprocessed) foods as possible.

4. Utilize the Glycemic Index to select foods. Consume a vast majority from the low glycemic category.

Institute gradual changes over time. 'Practice' will indeed make you 'perfect' at changing your habits until you have made 'permanent' improvements in your lifestyle of wellness.

A Solid First Step

A solid first step is necessary in order to set your direction and purpose toward any goal or destination—anything less results in misdirection and lack of focus. This philosophy applies to both life and business. In regard to life, I attempt to guide patients and clients using this philosophy as they make lifestyle changes toward the enhancement of their wellness. To that end, here are some tried and true principles to assist you in securing that 'solid first step':

Goal setting

1. Set short term and easily attainable goals at the outset. An example is setting a goal of 70 minutes of dedicated activity the first week. This goal can be achieved throughout the week in as little as 10 minute increments. Gradually increase your target activity minutes in the following weeks.

2. Set your goals with the mindset of 'guaranteed success.' This means your goals should be set realistic and 'failure proof.' There are too many failed goals in regard to wellness. We NEED to string successes together.

Nutritionally

1. Minimize the exposure around your house to foods that are high in saturated fat and low in nutritional value. Learn to read labels and educate yourself on food. A couple of great websites are www.myplate.gov or www.ultimatepaleoguide.com.
2. Utilize nutritional supplements to assist with nutrition. Supplements are NOT designed to replace food; they are designed to supplement where food does not deliver. I would like to see most of your nutrition come from food. However, since food quality is lacking, supplementation is necessary. Check out www.live4e. com for many of the quality pharmaceutical grade supplements I utilize daily.
3. We all eat out. However, choose to frequent places that provide healthy and tasty meals. Nearly every menu has options. Select a quality protein, quality fat, and low glycemic carbohydrates, and you cannot go wrong. You will be happy to know that food, as I describe in the previous sentence, does NOT have

to taste horrible. Remember, food is a fuel, it is not the engine.

Physically

1. Start a walking program. Take it slow and steady. Be consistent.
2. If your goal is to lose weight, target a 1 to 2 pound loss per week. This will ensure your maximum retention of lean muscle, which burns more calories and is much needed as we age.
3. A 5-10% reduction in bodyweight over a 6-month period provides benefits toward the reduction of cardiovascular disease, hypertension, and diabetes.

Friend, it is time to ignore the hype, avoid the fad, and take the 'solid first step.' Your life is important and is marked by each step you take.

PART 1

Physical Wellness

Activity /Exercise

1440 minutes—That is ALL You Get

We are all well-schooled and even inundated on concepts of financial management (e.g. "spend less—save more", "don't spend more than you make", "pay yourself first", etc.). How about the concept of time management? Do we really understand it? Do we practice, or are we even aware of, good habits in this area? I bring up this subject because I constantly hear the words, "I just don't have time to exercise." Let me make this statement to the readers, "YOU DON'T HAVE TIME TO NOT EXERCISE!"

Let me explain. Unlike finances, in which we can always earn more or less, time is a precious commodity with which we are blessed. We cannot produce more, but we can certainly increase our chances to have less. We would not even consider purposely increasing our chances to make less money; would we? Then why would we consider purposely increasing our chances to have less time? However, that does seem to be the case for some. If you have found yourself uttering the words above, "I just don't have time to exercise," this chapter is for you.

Each day, we are limited to 1440 minutes. That is ALL we get. The following principles regarding this concept are universal:

1. There is no more, but there could be less.
2. It is up to our own discretion on how we manage the minutes.
3. We can spend more or less on what we choose.
4. We cannot spend more than we make.
5. We can pay ourselves first.

I want you to place your focus now on number 5. You are blessed to be alive. You are blessed to have a body that is capable of functioning relatively efficiently and healthy. You should feel an obligation to pay yourself some of those precious minutes (on a daily basis) in order to show gratitude by caring for the life (and body) you are given. Let's face it; you can't afford to treat it badly, or it most certainly will not last long. I have never seen a trailer hitch on a hearse (i.e. "you cannot take it with you").

As those 1440 minutes per day in your life are assessed, do you spend them wisely or carelessly? One sure-fire way to add wisdom to your minutes-per-day budget is to force yourself to incorporate a sound, well-developed exercise program. I have not met a person yet who says that a consistent exercise program is not valuable. The problem rests in our lack of perspective regarding the 1440 minute limit of our day. We must begin and continue to exercise for the rest of our lives. We must treasure those valuable (limited) minutes. Pay yourself some minutes! Increase the likelihood of being blessed with more! You owe it to yourselves and those around you!

The Power of 10

"10" is a unique number. It has been used variously in our society including to describe perfection or indicate an expected percentage. In either of these contexts, the overlying theme is a targeted goal. Describing it better, I can say, "We will never be perfect but we can tailor our effort to reach a goal in a 'perfect' manner." Or, "We may not be able to give a lot, but '10'% is a great target (esp. regarding finances). Now, let's examine how this fits into our life from a broader perspective.

We may indeed never be perfect, but we can certainly give perfect effort. As a man with principles, I operate under the premise that if I give 10% of my income to the local church, I know (principle speaking) I will be blessed with more to give. Personally, I have seen that proved many times over during my lifetime. With that said, how about we target 10% of our daily time targeting our wellness? I have spoken before about the necessity to effectively manage each of the 1440 minutes we are granted daily.

Mark Sherwood, ND | 🐦

10% of 1440 minutes is 144 minutes. This roughly equals 2 hours and 24 minutes. By DEDICATING 10% of your total allotment of daily time to wellness, you will be blessed with MORE to give. Here is a simple guide on how to spend your 10%:

30 minutes–dedicate this to some sort of physical activity. Walking is always an option and is a very safe form of exercise. Studies have shown minimal amounts of walking lends itself to a longer life (refer to my article on this topic).

35 minutes–plan a meal during the day that is consistent with producing healthy results. The meal should consist of lean protein (fish, chicken, beef, etc.), vegetables, and a piece of fruit.

5 minutes–journaling your activity completed during the 30 minutes. What did you do and where?

35 minutes–eat another meal similar to the one described. By doing this again, you can ensure you are at least getting two meals a day of great quality.

15 minutes–spend this time talking with your spouse or significant other. This conversation is uninterrupted and void of distractions (no TV or cell phones allowed).

15 minutes–read a motivational or uplifting book. There are many out there from which to select. You should also incorporate my FREE 14 days to Freedom devotional (found on my website www.live4e.com).

9 minutes–use this time to be quiet. Do not allow interruption. This is often utilized first thing in the morning or late in the evening. It is critical to dedicate this time to

practice prayer, meditation, or simple intra-spection (e.g. How did I do? Can I improve?).

There you have it! 144 minutes (10%) guaranteed to be NOT WASTED TIME. Incorporate this plan in your life (or a form thereof), and you will see you time multiplied and blessed!

Can Exercising Increase Your Life Expectancy?

Lets ask the question WHY should we exercise?

In working with people across the world, I am continually met with the question in regard to physical activity, "What's the use?"

I feel compelled to address this head-on. First, the majority of large health organizations recommend, as a minimum, the following:

150 minutes of moderate exercise weekly–this can be as simple as brisk walking. OR 75 minutes of high intensity exercise weekly–this is defined as continual activity in a heart rate zone of 70-85% of your max. (NOTE: Max heart rate can be determined by subtracting your age from 220. The result is 100% of your max heart rate. You will then multiply that number by .70 and .85 to determine the range.)

Having stated the above, here are some relevant statistics to ponder...

- For each hour of moderate exercise, studies show an increase average life expectancy of 2 hours.
- For each minute of moderate intensity exercise, you will receive on average return on investment (ROI) of 1 to 7 (1 minute of moderate exercise = 7 additional minutes of life expectancy).
- For each minute of high intensity exercise, you will DOUBLE your ROI to 1 to 14 (1 minute of high intensity exercise = 14 additional minutes of life expectancy).

If that doesn't speak volumes to the "What's the use" question, maybe this will...

- If a person simply does the minimum recommended weekly amount of moderate exercise, one can add potentially 3.4 years to their life.
- If a person does twice the minimum recommended weekly amount of moderate exercise, one can add potentially 4.2 years to their life.
- If a person does EVEN HALF of the recommended weekly amount of moderate exercise, one can add 1.8 years to their life.

I trust the above-data provides pertinent information for you to consider. As we all realize, it is NOT just about the amount of life, but it is also about QUALITY. I assure you that by coming to the realization that exercise is a NECESSITY TO QUALITY OF LIFE, the "What's the use" question will never reach your lips again.

Life is never about being easy, but I am all about not adding difficulty. Employ and enjoy the ability to exercise. You will be happy you did.

The answer to the question is to Enjoy the journey…a little bit longer!

Physical Activity—a necessary and available resource

There is little argument that being active is healthy for both the body and soul. We just discussed how exercise can increase your quality of life and life expectancy. With obesity rates climbing along with parallel increases in health care costs, there is no time like the present to take a fresh look at how we can fit activity into our busy schedules.

Here are some tips to consider:

1. What do you enjoy? Walking? Running? Biking? If you enjoy something, it makes it easier to do on a regular basis.
2. What is the current state of your health? Have you had a recent check-up? If you are healthy, select an activity that is both fun (see #1) and safe.

3. Find a location in the community where others share the same activity.
   a. Examples:
      i. If you like running, find a park or track where others frequent.
      ii. If it is walking, many cities have community centers that are packed with walkers. Other great places are indoor malls or church gyms.
      iii. If it is an organized sport such as softball, tennis, golf, etc., there are many clubs found through a simple online, local newspaper, or local magazine search.
      iv. If it is weightlifting or group exercise, you can find a local gym or YMCA. Oftentimes, personal trainers offer group activities that meet in a parking lot or park.

It is time to eliminate excuses and search for solutions, which is a powerful and life-changing shift in mindset. The answers to the obesity crisis and increasing health care costs are not that complicated. We just have to DO SOMETHING about it. Let's be pro-ACTIVE in arriving at the solution. The following chapters are dedicated to topics on exercise. There is something for everyone. Pick a title that suits your needs and dig in.

From Contemplation to Action

We might want to get started but just can't get our feet moving into the right direction to exercise. The following steps can move you in the direction of success with your exercise or activity plan.

Recently, I read some information that indicated many persons are contemplating, or have contemplated, beginning an exercise program. Sadly, many of these same persons stay in the contemplation stage and never progress to action. We can 'say' all day that we 'need' to start an exercise program, but until we 'do,' nothing actually occurs. So, what does it actually take to move someone from contemplation to action?

First, we need to accept that all talk and no action equals empty words. Second, we must realize that by taking action, we will receive a positive reaction (better health). So, let's get to it. Here are some 'action' steps:

1. Write down some realistic goals...both short term (3 months) and long term (1 year).
2. Get with a trusted source, such as a personal trainer, to discuss your goals.
3. If they are agreed upon as realistic, develop a plan.
4. Sign a contract of agreement with your trainer regarding your commitment and accountability.
5. Begin execution of the plan at your first opportunity. Do not delay.

6. Revisit your goals on a weekly basis. Are you on track?
7. Realize that you may experience some setbacks such as a missed workout.
8. Cut yourself some slack if you do miss a workout and keep moving forward. Don't try to make it up.

Folks, now is the time to move from contemplation to action. I wish I had a dollar for every person that has said to me, "I know I need to start a program, and I am going to start one day." Make that 'one day' today. Your life and health is too valuable to wait any longer. It is ACTION TIME.

From Inactivity To Exercise

It seems this is a common theme today—"Where do I begin when it comes to beginning an exercise plan?" With so many options to choose from, I thought I would lay out some basic guidelines to follow when 'just starting out.' Please understand that when I say 'just starting out,' I am speaking to those who know they should exercise, have had many setbacks, and have not been doing much of anything. It may go without saying, but always make sure you are healthy and ready to begin a program. This may mean a visit to a doctor for a quick check up. The worst that can happen with this is that the doctor will confirm you're healthy.

It all begins with setting realistic and attainable goals. A couple of good examples of this type of goal may be:

1. Exercising at least 3 times a week for the next 2 weeks.
2. Doing some sort of cardiovascular activity at least 60 minutes per week for the next 2 weeks.
3. Actually going to a gym to exercise at least 2 times a week for the next three weeks.

You may notice one commonality with these ideas—they are all relatively simple and short-term. This design is so that a person will experience a quick success rather than certain failure. An example of a 'destined to fail goal' may be committing to visit the gym 5 times a week for the next 6 months.

Now that you have a goal, here is a good idea when it comes to cardiovascular activity. First, select an activity you enjoy—whether it is walking, running, biking, etc. Set an attainable goal of 'minutes of that activity' you wish to achieve during a week. Let's say you enjoy walking. A good goal may be to walk at least 60 minutes during a week. This would mean 30 minutes two times that week or 10 minutes six times that week. You get the idea! We are talking 'minutes per week' rather than 'per day.' Keep track of your 'minutes' in a journal. If you feel like walking more, that is great. However, just make certain that you set your initial goal LOW ENOUGH THAT YOU ARE CERTAIN TO SUCCEED. This is of utmost importance. After reaching your initial goal, set another slightly more difficult. Continue this process THE REST OF YOUR LIFE.

Additionally, prepare yourself for setbacks. No person is perfect. There will be some times in the future where you may fail to reach your goals. THIS IS NORMAL. Just cut yourself a break and keep looking ahead. Overall, however, you want to set your goals (especially early on) where there is little chance for failure.

Later in the process, you will want to shoot for an overall goal of doing some type of cardiovascular activity for 5-6 days a week (most weeks) for an average of at least 150 minutes per week. This will ensure you are getting a basic amount. Obviously, over time, you will want to increase intensity (effort, speed, time) to ensure continued progress and development.

At some point in this process, you will want to institute at least two days a week of resistance training (weight training). It is important to exercise and train the inner muscle (heart) and the outer muscles as well. This increases our chances of overall health. Resistance training can be accomplished in as little as two 30-minute sessions. For the development of a resistance training program designed specifically for you, seek out a professional trainer (or person of expertise). Don't just listen to what you may 'hear about.' This is risky business when we are talking about lifting weights. Every person is made a little different, so 'one size' does NOT fit all.

There you have it! This is no magic pill; just good old-fashioned hard work and consistency. Keep it up for a lifetime of healthy living!!!

❦ | Limitless Strength

Workout 101—Cover All the Bases

Very frequently, I am asked about my workout routine. The questions sound something like this, "What type of workout do you do? How can I get as big as you? How do you get so cut and stay big? What do I need to do to get bigger?" These are just a few. First of all, let me begin by saying that each of us is unique and specifically designed. You are you, and I am me. None of us should try to be someone else. It is impossible. We all need to be the best 'me' we can be! Though certainly, emulating others' desired characteristics is beneficial, we can never fully 'become' someone other than ourselves. Regarding the workout routine, there is one universal principle that we should always remember: COVER ALL THE BASES. This means training properly inside and out. In physical training, we must properly put attention to our cardiovascular system AND our muscular skeletal system. By adequately training BOTH, our workout routine is optimized.

So, let's get down to the nuts and bolts. Here is a great, basic routine that 'covers all the bases':

Aerobic (cardiovascular) training (I have outlined/defined this in a past article—see archives):

5-6 days a week for at least 20 minutes per session

Resistance (muscular) training:

2-3 days a week following this pattern:
Squats/Leg Press—5 sets of 10-12 reps

Bench Press—5 sets of 10-12 reps
Lat Pull Downs (to the front)—5 sets of 10-12 reps

Try to rest about 90 seconds between sets and rest at least 1 day before repeating this workout. Do not do it on consecutive days! The above may sound very simple and basic. However, by practicing the principles of progressive resistance (also outlined in previous articles—see archives) while getting proper rest, this workout will be extremely effective.

Folks, it is not rocket science! It is good old-fashioned hard work that is well-planned. Commit to this plan and give it a try for a couple of months. It 'covers all the bases' and will lead you down the path of living the 4E wellness life!

Balanced Training

It all breaks down to balance, staying balanced in all things including our training. If one thing gets out of balance it can lend a weak foundation and then there is really nothing to stand on.

Far too many times when I have visited gyms across this country, I have observed the following site:

A man in the far corner of the gym is sweating and grunting as he stares intently at the reflection of his chiseled upper body. His chest, arms, and shoulders are all visible as the only covering on the upper torso is a gray colored string tank top. The upper body muscles are bulging with amazing striated definition as other

❦ | Limitless Strength

gym occupants cut quick jaw-dropping glances. One can almost imagine what the onlookers are thinking…"I wish I had arms like that"…"I wonder how he got his chest that defined"…"How do I get those shoulders that are shaped like boulders?"

I notice that as his upper body is clearly visible while his lower body is covered by baggy, possibly oversized, pants. Something seems dreadfully wrong and out of place. It is one of those moments where you just know "something is not right." I just can't figure it out. After I complete my exercise session, I run into the Greek god looking man in the locker room. He looks much different now. I will not describe what he is wearing, but let's just say I can clearly see his upper body AND lower body. His upper body is still impressive. However, his lower body looks like a couple of thin brittle sticks underneath this massive upper body. We strike up a conversation at which time he mentions to me that he is getting ready to go on a jog "to work his legs." As the conversation continues, I quickly realize this man is like many others across this country. He believes he can train his legs for strength by jogging.

Jogging is an aerobic activity designed to work such things as the heart, lungs, and respiratory system. Jogging will NOT train the legs for strength. You must train your upper body and lower body with weights in a *balanced manner*. If the principles of resistance training are not followed for the entire body, imbalanced training will result. This, in turn, results in an imbalanced physique (e.g. a large upper body and a small lower body). An imbalanced physique is increasingly susceptible to injuries. Do not neglect the training of your lower body with weights, or flexibility training of the arms.

Balanced training **for a balanced physique is the answer.** Don't neglect the legs or any other part of your body. Train each part equally and in a balanced manner in order to prevent foundational weakness and create undue ground for injury.

Try This for Increased Arm Size

On more occasions than I can count, I have observed a recurring scene play out as I have conducted my daily workout routines. Have you ever seen (or been a part) of the following?

Two guys are in a section of the gym near a large section of wall mirrors. A large rack of assorted dumbbells is nearby. The men are taking turns curling these dumbbells as they let out exhausted "grunts and groans" while counting their repetitions. Between sets, they make statements such as, "My arms used to be bigger...I don't feel a pump yet...Let's do a few more sets." The "grunts and groans", repetitions, and comments continue for nearly one hour as the men try to stare and flex their arms into an approved size. The men then leave the gym exhausted while rubbing their biceps.

Unfortunately, these gentlemen's arms probably will NEVER be the size they want because they are training them TOO MUCH. The arms contain relatively small muscles compared to other parts of the body, namely legs, chest, and back. Because they are comparatively small, it does not make sense to train them MORE. Therefore, we need to train the muscles of the arm LESS for MORE growth. Yes, LESS is MORE!

The following arm routine (performed two times per week) will increase and provide much desired growth. Try this one on for SIZE:

Workout #1

Alternate these two: Machine Triceps pushdowns 3 sets (10, 8, 6 reps)

Dumbbell biceps curls 3 sets (10, 8, 6 reps)

Alternate these two: Triceps kick backs 2 sets (10, 8 reps)

Hammer curls (dumbbells) 2 sets (10, 8 reps)

Workout #2

Alternate these two: Dips4 sets (10, 10, 10)

Barbell curls4 sets (10, 10, 10)

Keep track of the weight you are using and continue to increase weight as you complete the listed reps with ease. The last set should be performed with difficultly in order to complete the last rep.

There you have it. LESS is MORE! This routine will prevent overtraining these relatively small muscles and initiate new growth. Try this workout and watch your arm size increase.

Heavy Weight Training

After more than two decades of being involved in the fitness industry, I have had much experience in assisting both men and women with resistance exercise plans. During this time, I have also had many of these same people (especially women) state to me, "I don't want to lift heavy weights and bulk up." The women further state at times, "I am afraid of looking like a man!" Let me alleviate this concern now by stating to women that you will NOT look like a man. Women do not need to fear this because of far less quantities of testosterone in their bodies. And for both men and woman…having more lean muscle mass is a great thing.

Heavy weight training, which I will define in a moment, is actually incredibly beneficial if done safely and correctly. This type of training not only facilitates growth of lean muscle, a critical element to increased metabolism and fat burning, but also stimulates increased density to the bones (more calcium and more stability). Heavy weight training, also known as high intensity-low volume training can be described generally as follows:

5-8 repetitions at 75-85% of your one rep maximum weight in which you can lift on a particular exercise. Here is an example:

Let's say your 1-rep max in the bench press is 100 lbs. 75% is 75 lbs., and 85% is 85 lbs. These 5-8 repetitions are

❦ | Limitless Strength

performed in 3-4 set intervals with 2-3 minutes of rest between each set.

I recommend both men and women, who have been involved in consistent (at least 3 times/week) resistance exercise for at least 3 consecutive months, add the following routine into their plan *2 times per week*:

Bench Press	3-4 sets	5-8 reps
Lat Pull downs (front)	3-4 sets	5-8 reps
Leg Press	3-4 sets	5-8 reps

All these are done at 75-85% of 1-rep max.

Mix in this type of training for 1 month at a time. Take a month off (return to higher repetition, lower weight training) before returning again to the heavier training. There is no need to fear "bulking up." The benefits you will experience are amazing. The only thing to "fear" is being leaner, feeling better, and being stronger.

Progressive Resistance— A Must for Growth (Part 1)

Throughout my 25 years of intense weight training, I have been asked numerous times for input on specialized workouts, training ideas, and of course, supplements. As you can guess I wholeheartedly and only endorse professional grade supplemental products. However, the purpose of this section is not about supplementation, but to give you **the "key" to increased growth and improvement in your weight training program**.

Let me begin by informing you of the *most common error* people can have in weight training. **It is doing the same old thing over, and over, and over again without adding/ increasing resistance**. This principle is clearly illustrated by the body's tremendous ability to adapt. Over time, our bodies will adapt to stressors (this can be internal or external changes). Without getting too complicated, this adaptation occurs when our body adjusts itself to believe the current situation (or stressor) is the norm. The body adapts so that it can handle the new norm with ease. To make this clear, I want you to imagine a 40 year-old male going to the gym 3 days per week and performing one exercise with the same weight and repetitions each time.

For example:

Every Monday, Wednesday, and Friday—our subject performs 3 sets of flat bench press (loaded with 135 pounds) for 10 repetitions. These three sets are performed after a proper warm-up with exactly 90 seconds of rest between sets.

Our subject performs this same exercise routine religiously for 6 months. To some, this may appear extremely effective and diligent. However, our subject's body *adjusted* to the stress of this exercise well before the 6 month period ended. He probably did improve his lean muscle mass for a time, but the potential for growth and improvement ceased after a few weeks. But why, you may ask.

Lean muscle mass is built by the tearing down, resting and recovery, and rebuilding process. When we lift weights, our muscles are broken down (or slightly torn apart). With proper rest, recovery of this slight destruction begins. The body is excellent at recovery. Therefore, after the rest and recovery period, rebuilding will occur. Here is where the brilliance of our body reveals itself. The body not only rebuilds the muscle back to its previous condition, but actually to a condition that is stronger than before. This is done so that we can handle the previously performed load with ease the next time we perform it. Back to our example above, the subject performs the 135 pound bench press, causing muscle breakdown, gets the proper rest and recovery, and has rebuilt muscle to perform the 135 pound bench press the next time. The body has a tremendous ability to remember the last stressor and adapt to handle it easier next time. The body no longer has to work as hard to perform the exercise…therefore less muscle tear down…resulting less potential rebuilt muscle.

I hope you are beginning to get a clearer picture now of the concept of **progressive resistance**. If we continue to perform the same exercise routines repeatedly, our bodies adapt easily to handle it. The need to develop more muscle is reduced because we haven't increased the resistance progressively (e.g. added a little weight to the exercise every so often). We all would love to have more lean muscle mass. It is a critical piece to our body's metabolism and its ability to burn fat. But, you cannot guarantee the potential for the increase in lean muscle until you understand the **principle of progressive resistance**.

So begin to add weight to your exercise incrementally and systematically over time. Document this in a training journal and begin to see your strength and lean muscle mass improve. More to come on this subject…

Progressive Resistance— A Must for Growth (Part 2)

As you recall, during part 1 of this discussion topic, I defined the concept of progressive resistance and how a clear understanding of it (put into practice) can effectively increase your body's lean muscle mass. The weight training example that served as our baseline was as follows:

Example:

Every Monday, Wednesday, and Friday—a person performs 3 sets of flat bench press (loaded with 135 pounds) for 10 repetitions. These three sets are performed after a proper warm-up with exactly 90 seconds of rest between sets.

As this routine is performed, it is necessary to continue to increase resistance (add weight) in order to continue to build more lean muscle mass. As you may have guessed, there reaches a point in time where the ability to add weight will slow. After all, if a person could continue to add weight, the upper limits of how much weight that could be lifted would be infinite. We know that is not true. There are limits to what each of us can eventually lift. Further, each of us (being different and unique) has a region of what I like to call "personal upper limits." The trick is to reach these "personal upper limits" as expeditiously and safely as possible.

But, what happens when you cannot add more weight? What is another key to keeping your lean muscle building potential in an optimum state?

There are three specific things you can do to find new baselines of weight in which you can incorporate the principle of progressive resistance.

1. Increase your exercise intensity by shortening the period of rest between sets (see example above) from 90 seconds to 60 seconds. This will lower the amount of weight you can lift (new baseline), but will increase the intensity of the exercise. Do not be discouraged by the lesser amount of weight in which you are performing the exercise. This increase of intensity will give your lean muscle building mission a boost. Trust me, you will feel and experience a new "burn" as your muscles are being primed for new growth.

2. Vary the speed in which you perform repetitions. By using the example above, you can do this by simply lowering the weight to your chest in a much slower

and controlled manner than your normal cadence. For example, you can lower the weight with a one-thousand one, one-thousand two, and one-thousand three cadence. Then, after lowering, explode the weight upward in a controlled routine manner. Again, the amount of weight you can effectively handle will decline. However, another baseline of weight is created from which you will build.

3. Change the main target exercise. This means (again using the example above) exchanging flat bench press with incline bench press, or by exchanging flat bench press with flat dumbbell press. There are a number of other exchanges you could do, but hopefully, you get the idea. You are still basically targeting the same muscle group, but performing a completely different exercise. When this is done, your baseline weights are again changed.

By utilizing the above methodology, you will ensure there are always things you can do to keep from becoming stagnant in your pursuit of increased lean muscle mass. I will stress to you that it is very important to document your exercise in a training journal. This way, you will remember what you did, see your progress, and continue the development of your lean muscle building plan.

Remember, progressive resistance works if properly understood and applied. It will produce consistent results.

❦ | Limitless Strength

Visualize it in your mind, believe it in your heart, see it happening, and achieve results!

Are You Doing Aerobic Activity or Just Kidding Yourself?

For the great majority of my life, exercise has been a major priority. I place it on the same importance level as eating and sleeping. In other words, it is necessary in order to live. Most of us realize there are two types of exercise: *aerobic and anaerobic*. In simple terms, aerobic exercise can be defined as "activity that elevates the heart rate on a continual basis and keeps it elevated over a period of time." Examples of this activity include running, bicycling, swimming, stair master, etc. Most experts agree, this period of time when your heart rate is continually elevated is generally said to be at least 10 minutes. Anaerobic activity can be defined as "activity that may elevate the heart rate but not necessarily keeping it elevated over a period of time." Examples of this activity include weight training, tennis, racquetball, sprinting, etc. Notice specifically the difference between the two activities: aerobic activity is clearly designed to maintain an elevated heart rate and anaerobic activity is clearly not designed to maintain the heart rate elevation. These are vast differences and should be remembered. Certainly, there is much more in depth explanation I could give for each, but this article will focus on the aerobic activity topic.

First of all, *I recommend conducting at least 5 aerobic sessions per week lasting 20-45 minutes for the rest of your life*. **It must be that important to you**. Specifically, the title of this chapter contains the question that you should honestly ask yourself. Within the following paragraphs, you will find keys to discover an accurate and truthful answer to this question. As we all know, (if we are alive) we have a heart rate. The heart rate is usually counted in the number of heart beats per minute (BPM). We need to understand two key components of our heart rate: *our resting heart rate and our maximum heart rate.*

Our resting heart rate can be obtained most accurately when you first awake and before you get out of bed. This can be done with a heart rate monitor or by simple utilizing a watch (with a second hand) and pressing a finger against one of the well recognized places on your body where you can feel the heart pumping: ex: the radial pulse on the underside of your wrist near your thumb, or the carotid pulse on the side of your neck in the soft spot in front of the sternocleidomastoid muscle. Using the watch method, simply find the "pulse" and begin counting the beats by ones (starting at zero) while you observe the second hand. Count the pulse for 10 seconds and multiply the result by six. Keep this number (your resting heart rate) in mind and check it often. At present, my resting heart rate is 48. This number can actually decrease over time as your aerobic fitness level improves.

One of the easiest ways to calculate your maximum heart rate is by subtracting your age from 220. My maximum heart rate is calculated as follows: 220 - 49 = 171. There are certainly other methods to calculate, but this will give you a good idea. OK, now for the extremely important information. Aerobic activity is generally optimized in the range of 65%–85% of your maximum heart rate. For me, the formula results are as follows: 171 X .65 = 111 and 171 X .85 = 145. Therefore, for me to actually do useful, constructive, and optimized aerobic activity, I need my heart rate *to be consistently between 111 and 145 BPM for at least 20 minutes.*

Trust me about this: most folks don't really pay attention to their BPM. They mistakenly believe that a nice leisurely stroll on a treadmill will accomplish the mission. Or possibly, slowly peddling on a stationary bike will ensure a daily necessary dose of aerobic activity. I am not saying these are bad. As a matter of fact, these are great starts. If you have not been doing activity on a regular basis, please start somewhere, even with a nice leisurely stroll around the block 3-4 times a week. We must treat activity as a necessary and critical piece of our ability to live.

I don't know about you, but I don't want to waste my time when I put the time out for exercise. I want (and expect) positive results. I know you do as well. So ask yourself the question, "Am I doing aerobic activity or just kidding myself?" Answer the question honestly with the previous information. If you need to make adjustments in your perceptions and beliefs about aerobic activity, do so. You will be glad you did. No one will know except you. If you don't know, there is possibly a chance this is the reason you are not as fit as you would like. It all starts with the very first step.

Exercise Maintenance— Does it really exist?

A colleague recently asked me a thought-provoking question regarding the concept of maintenance as it pertains to training. To maintain means to give attention to something to ensure it is in its proper working/functioning order. So, how do we properly train with our goal being to maintain?

To answer the question, let's establish a few things about our bodies. There reaches a point (most agree it is somewhere in the mid-20's) where your body begins to naturally lose lean muscle mass. Basically, this is simply the aging process at work. Once it starts, this loss of lean muscle mass continues each year until you die. Additionally, this lessening of lean muscle mass affects your metabolism in a negative way (meaning your metabolic rate declines). Metabolism is defined as the speed and ability in which your body burns food as energy. Isn't aging a wonderful thing?

With the decrease in lean muscle mass and the slowing of metabolism, we are in a situation of decline. This state of decline is combated in the following ways:

Limitless Strength

1. Progressive resistance (weight) training—to build lean muscle which in turn positively affects metabolism. I recommend a minimum of 2 resistance training sessions per week training all major muscle groups equally. The weight you use is relative. Just focus your training in the 10-15 rep range giving attention to form and control. Here is a great (and simple) 2 month plan:

- Do 3 sets of the exercises (one exercise at a time) in Week 1
- Do 4 sets of the exercises (one exercise at a time) in Week 2
- (Alternate in this manner for 2 months resting at least two days between resistance training sessions–we are focusing on good foundational structure and habits)

    Workout #1
    - (Rest 90 seconds between sets)
    - Select one–Bench press/Incline Press/Machine Press/Dumbell Press
    - Select one–Barbell Rows/Dumbell Rows/Lat Pull downs to front
    - Select one—Squats/Leg Press/Dumbell Lunges

    Workout #2
    - Repeat workout #1

2. Cardiovascular training—to increase cardio-respiratory fitness and burn body fat which positively affects metabolism. Start slow here and focus on

weekly 'minute' goals. Here is a simple plan to get you started (feel free to adjust the minutes—the idea is to be progressive through the 2 month period):

- ○ Week 1-80 minutes of activity (walking/jogging/ machine work)
- ○ Week 2 – 85 minutes of activity (walking/jogging/ machine work)
- ○ Week 3 – 90 minutes of activity (walking/jogging/ machine work)
- ○ Week 4 – 95 minutes of activity (walking/jogging/ machine work)
- ○ Week 5 – 100 minutes of activity (walking/jogging/ machine work)
- ○ Week 6 – 105 minutes of activity (walking/jogging/ machine work)
- ○ Week 7 – 110 minutes of activity (walking/jogging/ machine work)
- ○ Week 8 – 115 minutes of activity (walking/jogging/ machine work)

3. Proper nutrition—consisting of low-fat protein, quality monounsaturated and polyunsaturated fats, and quality carbohydrates in the form of fresh fruits and vegetables. This will help the body rebuild, have a steady supply of energy, and avoid storing excess fat.

With this established, I hope you can see how our definition of maintenance as it pertains to fitness must change. To maintain, we must steadily build at least as much as we lose. This building process requires steady attention, commitment, and dedication.

When you are already in a situation of decline, do not fall into the trap of thinking you can do the same things all the time (over and over again) and remain the same. Decline will occur. You must build, push, grow, and continue to pursue fitness in a proactive, aggressive, and progressive manner. Here's to increase instead of decline!

Training While Injured

Injuries!!! I hate them! Let's face it! Who likes to be injured? Whether it is a broken bone, torn ligament, ruptured disc, or a pulled muscle, an injury can cause major delays in your quest for wellness. They can bring discouragement and even depression. I suspect that as you're reading now, recollections of how you felt during your last physical set-back are becoming increasingly present in your mind. The question in which I am commonly is, "can I train while injured?" The answer is NOT a simple "yes" or "no." The answer is more to the tune of "probably" or "possibly."

Here is what I mean:

Obviously, if your injury has you totally incapacitated, training is not possible. Short of total incapacitation, there are options. For example, if you upper body is injured, you may be able to train your lower body and vice versa. Let's say you have a broken right arm, which I have had. The right arm is in a cast, but you can possibly do leg presses, leg extension, leg curls, calf raises, abdominal exercises (all for strength) while additionally training your cardiovascular system on a stationary bike or by walking. Let's say your left ankle is splinted for a sprain. You could perform chest press, arm curls, triceps extension, shoulder press, lat pull downs, abdominal exercises (all for strength) while additionally training your cardiovascular system on a hand bike. I hope you get the idea. Innovation is the key. Rather than get discouraged and depressed, "exercise" your mind through "innovative training ideas" and get to work.

Having an open mind and being willing to train while injured may indeed speed up your recovery and healing process. I will however, caution you with this. NEVER perform an exercise movement or begin a training program (while you are injured or not) without consulting with your doctor, surgeon, or specialist. You may indeed be surprised at what you CAN do.

The Most Insane Workout Ever— Guaranteed Results

With so many styles, types, and philosophies of workouts, it is no wonder I am often asked for advice on this topic. As a workout veteran of over 30 years, I have learned a few things.

❦ | Limitless Strength

So, for the first time ever, I am going to attempt to blend this vast experience into the greatest workout with *guaranteed results*. That's right! I *guarantee* you will see results in, get this...one week. I know this sounds a little out of bounds for me when I constantly harp on lifestyle, but I want to ensure people get quick results with the ultimate goal to perpetuate a life of confidence, quality, and wellness.

The One-Week Workout

- **Day 1**—Avoid all sugar. This is tough, but well worth it. It will take all the power and strength from your heart. This will push your fitness to the next level. Come on, let's do this!
- **Day 2**—Avoid sugar and dairy. No, this is not overtraining. This is what it takes to be a champion. You are a winner, aren't you? Dig in! Let's get this done!
- **Day 3**—Avoid, sugar, dairy, and caffeine. You are not a wimp, are you? What do you mean you can't do *one more rep*? I need to see your inner tiger roar.
- **Day 4**—Avoid sugar, dairy, caffeine, and alcohol. What do you mean you can't do this? You are not a quitter are you? Come on, let me see how much strength you can muster!
- **Day 5**—Avoid sugar, dairy, caffeine, alcohol, and processed/packaged foods. Now, we are getting

somewhere. I can see that fat burning right off you! You wanted to get rid of that spare tire didn't you? Get off your backside and let's get this done!

- **Day 6**—Avoid sugar, dairy, caffeine, alcohol, processed/packaged foods, and gluten. We are almost there, just one more day! Dig in and get tough. I need to see what you are made of!
- **Day 7**—Avoid sugar, dairy, caffeine, alcohol, processed/packaged foods, gluten, and…take a 30 minute brisk walk. Finish the last rep strong! You have worked too hard to quit now. Come on, let's finish this thing!

There you have it! The 7-day workout that will produce the results…*guaranteed!* You see friend, it is really about the nutrition much more than about the workout. You can stack any sort of balanced workout (even walking) behind great nutritional guidelines and you will get results. The workout gets far too much credit. If you really want to be a *workout beast*, see if you can do this one! This is what really separates the champions from the "wanna be". If you don't believe me, I challenge you to try it! If you have the courage and strength to succeed, you will thank me after completion because your health (and life) is much better.

Nutritional

Time—Want More?

I recently saw a cartoon depicting a doctor speaking with a slightly overweight patient. The caption of the doctor speaking read, "Would you rather exercise one hour per day or be dead 24 hours a day?"

To me, the correct option seemed obvious. To others, I believe the choice posed seemed a bit harsh. As I thought more about it, I realized this question is quite possibly being avoided by millions around the world! We are driven to succeed...make more money...own businesses...own homes...take vacations...retire early...live the good life! Though these are extremely desirable and important goals, I must say NONE of them will matter if you are DEAD!! For me, to dance around this issue would be to side step my passion. I cannot do it!!!

I care enough about you to tell you the truth. With statistical data across this country clearly showing obesity on the rise, the truth MUST be told. Obesity is in epidemic proportions. There are no arguments that obesity has negative short and long term health implications…not to mention the emotional effect (we will leave that topic for another day). I have actually seen reports stating obesity "will be" over 60% by the year 2025. How alarming and sad!! It DOES NOT have to be so. We can change this dire prediction, and it begins with you and me. The two main causes of obesity are improper nutrition and inactivity.

Please pay attention! We cannot be part of the problem any longer; we must become the solution. If you are DEAD, you cannot enjoy earthly success, wealth, businesses, homes, family, friends, and fellowship. Could I be any more clear? We have address BOTH the nutritional element and the physical piece. In addressing both of these issues and increasing your likelihood of more time on this earth, you must do two things:

1. Research proper nutrition. Put REAL foods in your body. Experience real results!
2. Research a correct and balanced activity (exercise) plan. Incorporate this plan into your daily and weekly routine. Enjoy the benefits!

Listen, if you want more time, I challenge you with all that I have within me! Feed your body correctly and get active! Let's increase our time together and enjoy success, health, wealth, and a longer, higher quality, life

❦ | Limitless Strength

Are You In "Wellness" Debt?

We have all heard, read, seen, and possibly experienced the pitfalls of overwhelming financial debt. After all, even our very own country is experiencing trillions of dollars of debt. Financial debt, if not addressed and dealt with, can lead to work, family, and health problems. You will probably search in vain for someone who would disagree with the last statement. We are bombarded with debt reduction seminars and self-help books. The general strategy is to identify the cause, stop the increase of debt, and begin to chip away at it one small step at a time. That being said, I want to introduce an equally dangerous type of debt…wellness debt.

Rather than come up with a definition, let's paint a picture of the development of this condition…

Here is how it can begin. Over time, you have neglected placing an emphasis on physical wellness (exercise and eating correctly). You have "talked it," but not actually "walked it." Excuses for not exercising and eating correctly have become rote and routine. You are able to verbalize them without as much as a thought. Fatigue begins to increase along with the reading on digital scales in the bathroom. Your ability to handle life's problems (stressors) has become somewhat decreased. You find yourself feeling pressure and being on edge more often. That once calm "you" has been replaced with someone you don't even like. You are depressed and filled with anxiety. On the outside, you glare at yourself in the mirror and realize the person staring back at you doesn't look as good (or as healthy and vibrant) as you like. You say to yourself, "I need to start exercising one day." You even reach the point of saying, "I am going to start a workout program next week." However, next week never does arrive. You have now acquired the condition called wellness debt.

I am not trying to depress you with this description. I am trying to get your attention and ask you to be honest with yourself. With over 40% of Americans being considered obese (30 pounds or more overweight) and stress-related illnesses on the rise, I think there is a strong likelihood that some who are reading this article at this moment may be in need of a reality check. Additionally please remember, you do not have to be obese to suffer from wellness debt. Some extremely unhealthy people, who have a ton of wellness debt, can look slim.

Is this you? Are you in a place of wellness debt? Have you built up a mountainous lack of attention to wellness? It can be insurmountable and overwhelming. However, there is hope. In much the same way a person would address financial debt, you can begin to address wellness debt. Here are some actions steps:

1. Be honest with yourself. Don't sugarcoat! Are you in wellness debt?
2. Force yourself to MAKE mandatory regularly scheduled times available that are solely devoted to exercise.

_❦_ | Limitless Strength

3. Gradually make more healthy choices in the foods you eat. Try to eat at least one healthy meal a day at first with increasing frequency over time.
4. Educate yourself about foods/vitamins/minerals/supplements.
5. Get with a trainer or friend to help you develop an exercise plan.
6. Make the plan realistic with small, short-term, goals.
7. Begin to chip away at the wellness debt until it is eliminated.
8. After the wellness debt is eliminated, begin to build wellness equity.

Give yourself an honest wellness assessment!! The time is NOW to get out of WELLNESS DEBT!

NOW is the Time for Wellness

Life today is characterized by high alertness, being on your toes, remaining vigilant, and always aware. This art of survival challenges survival itself and threatens our health over time. To that end, here are two brief tips that make wellness much easier:

1. 20 and 2
    Technological advancements have made life more efficient...and, more sedentary. Take the time to

stand up and move more. An easy way to incorporate this is with the '20 and 2' rule. For every 20 minutes of sitting, stand for 2. When you stand, work on posture—pulling your shoulders back, head straight and tall, and stomach pulled inward and back. This action will force core muscle activation and actually assist in the fat-burning process.

2. Available and visible
    Have healthy snacks and water 'available and visible.' Whether in your office or car, have a couple of healthy meal replacement bars, fruit, or trail mix handy. Additionally, keep a bottle of water always near. If it is 'available and visible,' trust me, you will eat it. If it is not 'available and visible,' you will eat something, but it may not be the best option. So, take the guess work out and prepare in advance.

Here's to making time NOW for wellness!

Solid First Step-Revisited

"I need to start exercising; I know that!" I hear these words literally every place I speak. It seems that even though many people are aware of the problem (i.e. obesity, sedentary habits, poor nutrition, and poor health are all on the rise), few take the steps necessary for correction. I really believe that most reasons for not taking those steps are found somewhere

❦ | Limitless Strength

between internal feelings of overwhelm, fears of failure, and uncertainty about where exactly to begin.

The first step is the most important. This step must be certain, sure, and solid. It cannot have question and must succeed. With 360 degrees of option in that first step, there are many choices of direction, but only a very few will get you going the right direction.

Ok, so here is a simple breakdown of a solid first step—4 simple guidelines everyone can do at a price everyone can afford:

1. Begin adding better nutritional choices to your diet. Make careful food selections and carefully research nutritional supplements. A good plan is very affordable and a foolproof way to put valuable nutrients in your body.

2. Make gradual changes to your diet. Start small by trying to add two servings of vegetables per day at least 5 days per week. Don't start worrying about taking things away just yet.

3. Drink more water. A good rule of thumb is to divide your body weight by 2 and drink at least that many ounces of water daily.

4. Begin a simple, structured, low-resistance strength, flexibility, and cardiovascular program at home. Don't try to visit a gym just yet. For a one-time price of $50, I recommend my 4E Fitness BASIC

and INTERMEDIATE DVD programs. They are affordable and very effective with amazing flexibility on when/where they can be used. Just pop them in a laptop or DVD player and follow along. A simple walking program is included.

For at least 6 months, follow these 4 simple guidelines that encompass the all important first step. You will have made that first step successful, solid, and sure. It will be time well spent and money well invested. It will change your life for the better. This is a price you cannot afford 'not' to pay. Your health is extremely important! Don't wait! Take that first step now—not tomorrow—but now!

We don't know what tomorrow holds, but we do have the chance to make the most of NOW. As you read this, please know that I believe in you, and I believe that this first step (described above) is a step in which you will be successful.

Help, I NEED to Lose a Few Pounds

I have been asked at least 100 times (if not 1000) how to lose a few pounds. Before addressing this topic head on, I want to establish a couple of things:

1. Scale weight is a symptom of behavior—either good or bad. If the scale weight declines because of

Limitless Strength

exercise and good nutrition, that is great. In others, proper exercise and nutrition can cause scale weight to increase. The opposite of each is true.

2. All weight loss is not healthy (e.g. if it involves malnutrition, a severe and rapid loss of lean muscle tissue, or artificially increasing your heart rate to 'give you more energy and need less sleep'). Starving yourself will cause catastrophic effects on your health at the sacrifice of much needed lean muscle tissue. Increasing your heart rate through artificial stimulants will cause overstimulation, which, over time will take a heavy toll on the body.

3. Being fat (yes, I used that word intentionally) is NOT a sign of wellness. Being overweight is a major issue. Let us not become deceived by believing 10-15 extra pounds are OK and just a normal part of life.

4. Maintaining a healthy weight (with corresponding healthy waist to hip ratio) is a lifetime job. It is not a job in that the work is drudgery. Rather, it should be viewed as the ultimate opportunity to care for and maintain the unique gift we have been given...the gift of life in the human body.

Now to give you the answer to the question at hand...Here are a few things to assist with not only 'losing a few pounds,' but to keep up on the path toward optimum wellness:

DO:

1. Eliminate the use of sugars and processed or refined foods and grains.

2. Cut down on the things that bring your great stress. Set healthy boundaries. If something or someone drains the life out of you, a good pruning is in order.

3. Eat as natural as possible. Purchase raw as much as possible and cook your meals as often as feasible.

4. Use proper nutritional supplementation where deficient. Your practitioner or nutritional expert will help with this.

5. Drink plenty of water. Start with at least 1/2 ounce for each pound of body weight.

6. Walk or do some sort of cardiovascular related activity at least 150 minutes per week.

7. Use a pedometer and target 10,000 steps per day.

8. Maintain a resistance training program at least 2 days a week. Get with an experienced personal trainer for development and design. Anything less could produce injury and discouragement.

9. Practice yoga, meditation, or prayer.

10. Make the commitment to a lifetime of wellness. It is not a temporary thing to 'try,' It is something we have the 'opportunity to do' for the remainder of our days on earth.

11. Avoid falling for the 'quick fix' trap. Hard work, commitment, and consistency produce results.

| Limitless Strength

12. Avoid over spending and/or out spending your income. Debt will certainly bring destruction in your life.
13. Practice charitable giving of your time and money.
14. Get a full check up from a doctor who focuses on total wellness as opposed to treating symptoms.
15. Get at least 7-8 hours of sleep nightly. A warm shower or bath, soothing music, or reading a book prior to sleeping will help.
16. Take inventory. Make it a regular daily routine to evaluate your ability to follow good habits. Life requires discipline. When we continually take a look at where we are off track, it makes it easier to get right back on track.

DON'T:

1. Don't forget to follow 1-16 above!!! If you DO 1-16, you will always be guaranteed to 'lose a few pounds' and live a lifetime in your optimum state of wellness.

There you have it; the answer to the often-asked question, "how do I lose a few pounds." This may look so simple and easy…and it really is. We are not meant to walk this earth in a chronically unhealthy state. The sign of a few extra pounds is a sure sign of unhealthiness within, which will lead to more sickness and disease. LET TODAY BE THE FIRST DAY OF THE REST OF YOUR LIFE…a life of freedom, wellness, happiness, and health.

Get Rid of the Scales

It seems these days that there are so many issues surrounding weight and weight loss. If you don't weigh a certain number of pounds, you may consider yourself overweight or even fat (I don't like using that word, but let's be real). Further, if you view yourself as weighing too much, you may consider getting on some crazy weight loss plan. There are weight loss television shows, weight loss diets, weight loss drugs, weight loss doctors, weight loss witchcraft (well, maybe not that one). Folks, it is everywhere. What really saddens me is that weight issues seem to be a major source of depression and discouragement. In my day to day life, I have people tell me they are so discouraged about their weight that they don't even try at all. They are totally defeated in their attitude. This SHOULD NOT BE.

Let me just clarify a few things and give you some information to chew on. 5 pounds of muscle is approximately 1/3 smaller in actual size than 5 pounds of fat. What that means is that "weight" is a relative term compared to actual size. I am encouraging people all over the world to STOP using the scales as the sole motivator. It is literally causing people to lose weight at the sake of losing valuable lean muscle tissue. Did you know that lean muscle tissue naturally declines as you age? Did you know that lean muscle tissue actually assists in increasing metabolism?

❦ | Limitless Strength

Here is what you and I and EVERY single person across this world should seek: A positive change in body composition. This is described as increasing lean muscle tissue and decreasing fat. The way to get this accomplished is simple. Engaging in a sensible exercise plan (resistance and cardiovascular training) while being reasonable with your nutritional intake is the key. However, excuses seem to reign (time, job, family, church, motivation, location, knowledge, etc.). I have heard ALL types of excuses.

Unless you are faced with a very unusual circumstance, you have control over your own life. Yes, YOU!! You have the power to change things. It is time to see YOU in a different way. Let me encourage you with this:

You are unique and special. You are not designed for defeat and failure. You are not made to be depressed and down. You can achieve what you can believe. Scales no longer need to be your motivator. YOU need to be YOUR motivator. Be encouraged and driven from the inside. Commit to change your body composition so that the quality of your life (internal AND external) will improve.

I believe in YOU!!

You are NOT Meant to Be Fat

Whether you believe you evolved from an amoeba or were created by God (as I believe), you were not designed to carry excess fat to the point at which your health is increasingly poor and the likelihood of disease is great. I am not talking about a few extra pounds here and there that accumulate with age and a slowing metabolism. I am talking about the over-indulgence in poor food choices and habitual inactivity. Believe it or not, I have actually heard people say, "God made me like this (referring to a very obese state)." "You just need to love me and accept me the way I am."

Let me respond bluntly! I DO love people and DO accept them. However, I do not believe God made people obese, sick, and lazy. People are made with legs to walk and arms to move. Legs were not just designed to hang from a chair or lay limp on a couch. Arms were made for more than playing on a computer or iPhone.

We are designed to use our brain for reason/thinking and our bodies for movement. Do not allow yourself to be deceived. Wake up! The only person you are hurting (and badly I may add) is YOU. Don't make excuses because excuses hold you back from where you need to go. Excuses lock you down in a state of inactivity and denial.

You are not meant to be fat. You are designed for movement and activity with the purpose being to have a high quality of life while experiencing joy and happiness.

Foundational Eating—
Removing the Guesswork

With so many diet plans out there, I thought I would bring some sense and clarity to our chaotic inundation of these plans. First of all, let me cover some basics. Our body needs proteins, carbohydrates, and fat. We should get the majority of these through our food intake. Any diet plan that insinuates that you totally eliminate any of these is inherently flawed. There are some easy ways to identify types of food. By way of simple education, if something has/had a mother, it is probably mostly protein. If something came from a tree or the ground, it is probably mostly carbohydrate. It is important to note that most foods have some of each: protein, carbohydrates, and fat.

The key to a proper diet is two-fold: balance and quality. Balance refers to eating in moderation in reasonable portions. 3-4 smaller meals a day consisting of a good balance of protein, low to moderate glycemic carbohydrates, and quality fat is a great start. Here is a trick: Divide your plate into halves. On 1 half, you have your protein source. In the other half, you have your low to moderate glycemic vegetables and fruits. Go to www.live4e.com and print off the glycemic index for help. This dinner plate picture depicts balance.

Quality refers to the actual composition of each part. Quality proteins consist of lean cuts of beef, turkey, chicken, and fish. We do want to avoid fried food when possible. Quality fats consist of monounsaturated and polyunsaturated sources. You will want to minimize/avoid saturated and Trans fats. Quality carbohydrates consist of low to moderate glycemic vegetables and fruits.

As previously stated, supplementation is necessary in order to fulfill the quality component. These days, with a massive amount of processed foods available, you will want to put a little study and effort into the area of quality. It does not have to be so incredibly complicated. The bottom line is BALANCE and QUALITY. Do yourself a favor and simply follow these basic principles. These are foundational in nature and will help take a lot of the guess work out of it. As you get better at mastering these, you will want to build on them with study and education. Here's to balanced and quality eating!

The 14-Day Meal Plan: How to Effectively Give Up Old Eating Habits

When prescribing lifestyle alteration plans, I am often met with statements such as, "I am gonna have a hard giving up some of the things that I am used to eating. I know they are bad for me, but I really enjoy them." How many of you have uttered these words? Trust me, they are very, very common. With that said, let me identify what I call the BIG THREE. The big three are: sugar, bread, and dairy. As you probably noticed, the big three are very common in the standard American diet (SAD). It really boils down to eating too much of each.

❦ | Limitless Strength

We need a strategy targeting a reduced consumption of each without going straight to the 'cold turkey' approach. So here is a sound, reasonable, and novel plan for you to employ over a 14 day period (this will simply require a little bit of label reading):

The 14-Day Meal Plan

Day 1	Eliminate sugar (still eat bread and dairy)
Day 2	Eliminate bread (still eat sugar and dairy)
Day 3	Eliminate dairy (still ear sugar and bread)
Day 4	Eliminate the BIG THREE totally
Day 5	Eliminate sugar (still eat bread and dairy)
Day 6	Eliminate bread (still eat sugar and dairy)
Day 7	Eliminate dairy (still ear sugar and bread)
Day 8	Eliminate the BIG THREE totally
Day 9	Eliminate sugar and bread (still eat dairy)
Day 10	Eliminate bread and dairy (still eat sugar)
Day 11	Eliminate sugar and diary (still eat bread)
Day 12	Eliminate the BIG THREE totally
Day 13	Mardi Gras day (eat whatever you like)
Day 14	Eliminate the BIG THREE totally

As you can see by the aforementioned plan, during the 14 days you will have experienced 4 days of total elimination of the BIG THREE. Even though this plan is simple, it is very effective for two main reasons:

1. It requires more awareness of what we are putting in our mouths. This awareness is the first real step in making permanent lifestyle change.

2. We have given our body a 4 day break from three of the main food groups that plague our current lifestyle challenge. Your body will love it, and you will feel the difference. When you experience the better feeling, you will want to repeat the cause.

Try this plan today and begin to get free from food addiction. *The Wellness Life* is attainable for everyone,—all you have to do is start. **How about starting today?**

The True VALUE in a Meal

When we speak of value in regards to food, we are normally talking about a lot of food for little money. However, I believe we should consider in the equation the 'value' of the food itself. Is it quality and will it bring you nourishment? After all, nourishment is the REAL PURPOSE of food. With that said, allow me to outline a true value meal.

❦ | Limitless Strength

First, in this crazy world, we must speak of convenience. Therefore, I will take the 'fast food' approach to this subject. What I mean is this–I will discuss and compare those things we can obtain in less than 5 minutes. Further, I will denote the nutritional information of the compared 'meals.' Let's begin with a general comparison:

1. Arby's roast beef sandwich (classic)–cost $3.19
    360 calories (calories from fat 130)
    fat–14 grams (saturated fat 5 grams)
    carbohydrates–35 grams
    protein–23 grams
    sugars–6 grams
    (*source–corporate website*)

2. McDonald's cheeseburger (quarter pounder)–cost $3.79
    520 calories (calories from fat 240)
    fat–26 grams (saturated fat 12 grams)
    carbohydrates–42 grams
    protein–29 grams
    sugars–10
    (*source–corporate website*)

3. Functional Medical Institute's 'value meal in a glass'– cost $5.80
    Silk unsweetened almond milk (2 cups)–serving .75
    Cool processed whey protein (1 scoop)–serving $1.63
    Unflavored organic greens (9 grams–1 tablespoon)–serving $1.66
    L-Glutamine powder (3 grams–3/4 teaspoon)–serving .50

Vitamin C powder (3 grams–1 teaspoon)–serving .44
Unflavored fiber powder (5 grams–2 teaspoons)–serving .82
255 calories (calories from fat 65)
fat–7 grams (saturated fat 1 gram)
carbohydrates–15 grams
protein–28 grams
sugars–4 grams

After a general comparison of the three, let's go a little deeper... Notice the amount of saturated fat and the inflated amount of carbohydrates in item 1 and 2. Also, examine the amount of calories from fat in the total serving. Things are getting very interesting now! Look even closer... What about the quality of the actual ingredients? I will not go into inflammatory detail in regard to quality, but let me ask you this question–Do you believe the quality of meat in item 1 and 2 is of high quality? In comparison to the protein in item 3, which is sourced from organic, cool processed, grass fed beef, which is more beneficial for you?

In the 'value meal in a glass' we have added organic greens (for unsurpassed antioxidant protection and nutrient density). There is little argument we do not obtain enough of these in the Standard American Diet (SAD). We have also included glutamine and fiber for stomach repair and GI health. Face it; GI health is a big one today and is getting much more attention as understanding of it's relationship to overall health grows. Vitamin C has been loaded to generate much needed immune system support.

Pay close attention to what you eat. What is really promoting value?

Is it REALLY good for you?

Quality Protein—Where Art Thou?

In this day and age, everyone is talking about protein. Wherever I go on my travels, I am asked routinely two questions:

1. What kind of protein do I use?
2. How much protein should one consume?

Before I answer these questions, let me preface by saying I will be addressing this from a protein supplement standpoint, not food.

When selecting a quality protein, here are a few things in which to look. A quality protein supplement consists of: a source that has a high biological value, is very complete in its amino acid profile, is non-denatured-native (i.e. very low processed and as close to its original state as possible), and easy to digest and assimilate. Some examples of this include: year-round grass fed, non-denatured, low heat processed whey protein concentrate, miceller casein (a great non-denatured, slowly digested protein source), egg white or whole egg powder. There is also beef protein concentrate, but it can be difficult to stomach because of the taste. I utilize a non-dairy pea protein at times as well. This protein is created using organic non-GMO yellow peas. It is often (absent any allergic responses) a good idea to alternate the types of protein you use to keep your body on its toes. These proteins can be alternated by day, week, or bi-monthly.

Here are a couple of sure fire signs to know you may NOT be getting the best protein supplement: If the number one protein source in the product is soy concentrate or isolate, sodium caseinates, wheat protein (which is basically gluten!), these would be products to strongly avoid. Also, avoid very low cost whey protein products. They are likely produced from poor quality sources. These may be inferior quality protein sources at best, and at worst, may actually cause health issues with certain individuals.

In case you wondered, my choice of protein is non-denatured, year-round grass fed, and low heat processed whey. You would serve yourself well to incorporate this great tasting and high quality protein into your nutritional habits. You can read about in on my websites www.live4e.com or www.fmidr. com under online store.

In determining how much protein in which to use, I utilize the following formulas based on my most recent research (obviously these would be used ABSENT any unusual issues as diagnosed by your personal physician, nutritionist, or dietician):

If you practice a light level of activity (dedicated exercise less than 3 times weeks and very infrequently), multiply your body weight by .6. Your answer equals the number of grams of protein needed per day spread throughout 4-5 meals.

If you practice a moderate level of activity (dedicated exercise at least 3 times weekly for the past three months), multiply your body weight by .8. Your answer equals the number of grams of protein needed per day spread throughout 4-5 meals.

If you practice a high level of activity (dedicated exercise more than moderate), multiply your body weight by 1.0—1.2. You answer equals the number of grams of protein needed per day spread throughout 4-5 meals.

There you have it…probably more than you wanted to know.

Strategies for Reducing Saturated Fats

- Select lean cuts of beef and pork and limit portion sizes.
- Reduce consumption of butter and stick margarine.
- Reduce consumption of fried fast food.
- Reduce consumption of pastry or other baked goods.
- Reduce consumption of whole milk dairy products (unless natural and organic).
- Remove skin from chicken and turkey before cooking, select white meat.

Strategies for Reducing Sugars

- Avoids foods containing high fructose corn syrup, sucrose, fructose and any artificial sweeteners. This is especially true when one of this is listed as one of the first ingredients.
- Eat half or less your normal dessert portions.
- Use stevia or truvia as sweeteners rather than sugar or artificial sweeteners.
- Pay careful attention to drinks that are high in sugar...particularly alcohol.

Taming the Insulin Animal

We often hear about the dangers of elevated and abnormally high blood pressure and BMI (body mass index). Abnormal readings in the aforementioned do indeed promote cause for alarm. Action should be taken to lower each in order to minimize the risk of developing a dangerous health condition. As dangerous as each of these are, it is important to note an underlying cause in the elevation of each...that being the insulin animal. The insulin animal is much like a gerbil on a wheel. Once it gets set in motion it starts to spin faster and faster with greater and greater intensity until it spins out of control and burns itself out.

It has been said in ancient texts that "your enemy prowls around like a roaring lion seeking those he may devour." This wild beast of an enemy to our body is the hormone insulin. If insulin is continually elevated, our body is 'signaled' to store fat. The extra fat, in turn, can promote an increased BMI and negative body composition change (a little more belly fat being present). The extra fat taxes the body's system going so far as to cause an increase in blood pressure. So how does one tame this insulin beast and prevent the constant (and dangerous) elevation? The answer lies in understanding what makes it rise in the first place.

Insulin is triggered by the presence of glucose in the blood. Glucose is originally formed as a conversion product of carbohydrates. Carbohydrates, as you recall, are generally those foods that spring from the ground or grow on a tree. When carbohydrates are ingested, they are converted to glucose (simple sugar), a source of 'potential' energy for the body. As soon as the glucose is formed, the hormone insulin is released from the pancreas. Rapid influx of glucose (simple sugar) or large amounts in turn, release rapid and large amounts of insulin. It is important to note that the energy 'potential' in glucose is only 'potential' until it is ushered into the cell. The process of the cell receiving the glucose is only possible with the presence of insulin. Therefore , it can be said that insulin and glucose are 'two peas in a pod' and are an inseparable couple to facilitate the cell receiving the glucose making the energy 'potential' into energy 'reality.'

The problem of insulin being on constant elevation begins with the types of carbohydrates we eat and how quickly they are converted to glucose and the amount of insulin that the carbohydrate needs in order to be ushered into metabolic cells. It just makes sense that slowing down the conversion speed and rate of absorption from the digestive tract will slow down the insulin surge. The rate of insulin response in relationship to a specific carbohydrate is called the glycemic index. There is a printable version here http://live4e.com/gi. The glycemic index is the amount of insulin that each specific carbohydrate demands for its usage. Every carbohydrate is unique and does not relate to the carbohydrate being simple or complex. The use of a glycemic index chart lends you the ability to get a handle on taming the insulin animal. The goal is to keep the glycemic index of a carbohydrate in the low to low/medium range. A glycemic index chart is depicted with a 1 to 100 score for the insulin response to the type of ingested carbohydrate (The higher the score—the larger the insulin animal gets). Carbohydrates are generally listed in three categories of glycemic response—low, medium, and high. A quick example is the instant potato with an index of 84 (high) and a sweet potato with an index of 53 (medium). Obviously, the sweet potato would be the better choice. I could list other examples, but you get the idea.

Focusing on consuming low to low/medium glycemic carbohydrates is of utmost importance. To further give you

❦ | Limitless Strength

ammunition to not just tame, but defeat the insulin animal, incorporate the following:

1. Consume mainly low to low/medium glycemic carbohydrates.
2. Limit consumption of high glycemic carbohydrates.
3. Limit carbohydrate consumption to 30 grams or less per meal.
4. Stop all carbohydrate consumption at least 4 hours prior going to sleep for the night.
5. Set your carbohydrate goal in the sweet spot of fat burning- between 50-150 carbohydrates a day.

As you can see, my encouragement is to defeat insulin animal once and for all. These subtle changes I have outlined above will plant your feet firmly on the pathway to health and promote the reduction of metabolic crisis, excess body fat and other health destroying effects such as high blood pressure.

The Great Grain Giveaway

As I have crisscrossed the country, I have noticed a common theme in our restaurants and cafes. I like to call this "the great grain giveaway." People seem to like the free bread and/or chips, so restaurants have certainly obliged with the focus on drawing more patrons. It seems so normal now that wherever you go, there is a set expectation to receive a free grain product. Consequently, when I speak to folks about nutrition, I hear the dreaded questions/statements, "Do I have to give up my chips and salsa? I thought salsa was pretty good for you. I have to quit bread? It really fills me up."

Here is the down and dirty truth about this very common habit of ingesting free grain products...

Let's begin with the glycemic index (GI). The GI is a numerical scoring system (normally 1-100) to show how much glucose appears in the blood after eating a carbohydrate-containing food–the higher the number, the greater blood sugar response. A low GI food causes a small rise where a high GI food causes a dramatically higher spike. Most grade the scale with the following scale: 70 or more is high, 55-69 is moderate, and 54 or below is low. Consistently eating foods in the high GI category will most certainly lead to obesity, heart disease, and diabetes.

With that said, you will find it hard to swallow (I really mean that literally in a sense) that white bread is actually higher on the GI index than table sugar. Even wheat bread classifies as a high GI food. And corn chips...certainly they are high GI foods as well (not to mention a host of other very dangerous preservatives and chemicals).

Additionally, we probably most likely agree that "the great grain giveaway" is mostly enjoyed in the evening, a time in which we should be drastically reducing ALL carbohydrate consumption. As you can see, we have a huge cultural problem.

You might ask if the old Food Pyramid, suggesting we eat multiple servings of wheat and grain products, is meaningless. Let me simply say, "It was flat out in error and did not serve our nutritional or health needs well." Examine the steady rise in our obesity rates and we must come to the conclusion that the multiple serving of grains are NOT WORKING for us.

If you do choose to eat grains, see out sprouted grain (e.g. Ezekiel Bread), rye kernel, oat bran, or pumpernickel breads. These are all considered low GI foods. Avoid the chips all together. If you will utilize the glycemic index and stick with foods in the low to moderate GI categories, you will see beneficial (possibly astounding) results in your health.

Alcohol–What's the harm in a few drinks?

In my over 2 decades in the wellness industry, I have seen more than one of my colleagues and friends overtaken by the powerful effects of alcohol consumption. What may have begun as 'just a drink or two with work mates' became a powerful addiction that ended with a slow, torturous death. So is there anything really wrong with having a drink or two? The answer to that question is, "it depends." I believe in giving as much information as possible so that we can all make the best decision regarding alcohol consumption.

With that said, let's look at some effects of alcohol on the body and the desire to lose weight:

Effects of alcohol on the body's system

- Alcohol moves quickly through the body. It enters the blood without being metabolized in the stomach. Alcohol can be measured in the blood within 5 minutes of having a drink, and within 30 to 90 minutes after you've had a drink, the alcohol in your bloodstream will be at its highest level. The liver is responsible for most of the breakdown of alcohol once it is in your body. However, the body needs time, and if you are drinking alcohol faster than your body can break down the alcohol, the excess begins to move through your body and into other areas, such as the brain, where it can destroy cells.

Alcohol and the risk of hypoglycemia

- When a pre-diabetic person (many are without realizing it) consumes alcohol, he or she is susceptible to hypoglycemia, an abnormally low blood glucose level. Hypoglycemia can cause seizures, unconsciousness and in rare cases, brain damage or death.

Effect on diabetes

- Focusing on lifestyle changes is necessary to help ward off diabetes. If you are drinking, strictly limit yourself or stop altogether. You may safely consume a drink on occasion, depending on the severity of your pre-diabetic state. However, don't over-consume, and always allow your body plenty of time to absorb the alcohol. Alcohol raises HGa1C levels, which is a marker for pre-diabetes and a marker in the management of diabetes.

Alcohol and calories

- Aside from the effect on sugar production and metabolism in pre-diabetic persons, alcohol is a source of calories. Excessive intake of alcohol contributes to weight gain, which can in turn disrupt blood sugar levels. There are 7 calories per gram of alcohol, a fact that is rarely thought of in regard to its intake. One drink can lead to two, two drinks lead to three, and so on.

Commonsense prevention

- First, speak to your physician about alcohol in your diet to help reduce your chances of developing diabetes. If you do have a drink, make sure you aren't drinking on an empty stomach, and limit consumption to one drink if you are female, two if you are male. Select drinks that are low in alcohol and sugar, such as a spritzer. Also, use mixers that are sugar free, such as diet drinks, tonics, and seltzers or water.

Effects on weight loss

- If you need to lose weight, avoiding alcohol is a wise decision. Not only is alcohol packed with empty calories and devoid of any nourishment, but it is inhibiting your fat-burning AND fat-storing hormones, providing a double and triple whammy against all your weight loss efforts. If that's not bad enough, it lowers your inhibitions and changes your decision-making processes, causing you to make poor food choices. As stated, alcohol lowers your blood sugar levels, thereby making you feel hungrier and much more likely to consume excess calories. Add this to the calories from the alcohol, and you'll quickly see how bad alcohol is for weight loss. It makes loosing those extra pounds even tougher.

Other significant factors:

- Even worse, when your body is attempting to metabolize alcohol and food that have been consumed together, it will use the energy from the alcohol first and store the food as fat. Because the body perceives alcohol as a poison and because it cannot store the energy from alcohol, its first priority is to eliminate it, while digesting and processing the food becomes secondary. That means your meal gets stored and synthesized as fat while the alcohol

❦ | Limitless Strength

gets burned off. Because the food you've consumed is being stored and not properly metabolized with the overconsumption of alcohol, the nutrition from that food is not being absorbed by your body. The vitamins and minerals you need to be healthy are not utilized. Without adequate nutrition, your body is less healthy and more likely to store fat. Bottom line…too much alcohol causes insulin resistance and increase the likelihood of weight loss resistance.

Hopefully now, we all can make better decisions regarding whether or not to have that 'routine' drink after a hard day at work.

Detoxification—a Necessity for Optimum Wellness

The word detoxification brings on many shrugs of the shoulders and strange misunderstandings. The methods of detoxification, referring to the human body, do not mean using a laxative or cathartic to expel unwanted waste. Instead the word detoxification is an essential process that happens in many organs in the human system in order for the machine to keep functioning at optimal capacity. There are four main organs of detoxification, with the skin being the largest. The other three organs of detoxification, which cannot be seen from the outside, are the liver, kidneys and bowel. All of these organs have special functions to rid the body of waste on a moment to moment basis.

Our daily life can be toxic. From the air we breathe to the food we eat. Our organs of elimination have to be on duty to eliminate and get rid of anything that could disrupt its vital life line (the blood stream). More than 6 billion pounds of chemical pollutants are released into the air per year. Over the course of a lifetime, our bodies are exposed to thousands of foreign compounds via the food we eat, the air we breathe and directly through our skin. The degree of exposure determines the degree to which the organs of detoxification are called to eliminate or detoxify

When we eat, food enters the body. We don't think of what we eat as toxic, but perhaps we should. Everything that passes the tongue has to be evaluated, screened and either utilized to work (make more cells, energy, or other vital processes), stored for later use or eliminated. It is the organs of detoxification that do the work of elimination. The organs of elimination (detoxification) are then 'on-demand' to eliminate waste and unwanted goods as fast as they can. If these organs get bogged down, the system becomes slow or sluggish, hence the term "TOXIC". Toxins can derive from chemical pollutants, drugs, alcohol, cigarette smoking, food additives and preservatives. Toxins can also come from normal metabolism and an imbalance of unhealthy bacteria in the intestine. The Gastrointestinal system gets broken down with the Standard

❦ | Limitless Strength

American Diet lending it susceptible to bacterial imbalances and leaky gut syndrome. The weaker the gut, the more likely signs and symptoms of being toxic are present. The signs and symptoms of being toxic range anywhere from fatigue, body aches, pains, slow mental processing, heart palpitations, gut dysfunction and being overweight.

You can reduce your risk for toxicity and improve your body's ability to detoxify by following a few simple guidelines.

- Decrease the number of foods that cause ill health effects. Commit to a lifestyle of healthy eating and good nutritional habits. Avoid high trans fat/ saturated fat foods. Avoid eating vegetables that are overly sprayed with pesticides and coated in wax.
- Eliminate self-destructive behaviors such as cigarette smoking and excessive alcohol and taking drugs. Even too many over the counter medications have ill health effects and can cause metabolic burden. Get the help you need to break these health destroying strongholds. Cessation programs and counseling are both viable.
- Exercise on a regular basis. The skin, for example, eliminates waste through evaporation and perspiration. A simple walk in the park aids the system in clearing itself of metabolic sluggishness and pollution that may be hanging around in the blood stream or stored in body fat.

- Drink plenty of water. I recommend ½ your body weight in ounces of water per day. When we drink plenty of water, we aid the system of detoxification by dilution. One solution to pollution is dilution. Getting plenty of water every day aids elimination through a number of ways. Water improves perspiration and sweating through the skin. If we sweat more, waste hangs around less. Drinking sufficient water aids the kidneys, liver and bowel in their processes of elimination and detoxification. Water, first and foremost, is the simplest element of detoxification and elimination.

It is good to know you body is made to remove toxins. As a matter of fact, the term detoxification refers to our body's natural ability to transfer and eliminate toxins. To accomplish this, your body has to transform toxic substances into water soluble substances in order to effectively excrete them through the organs of detoxification. Toxic compounds are typically stored as fatty molecules and do not mix well in water. The detoxification process performed by the gut, liver and kidneys transforms these toxic, fat soluble substances into harmless, water soluble molecules which can then be excreted out of the body.

There are three phases of detoxification: The liver handles two phases of them. The liver will convert fat soluble toxins into intermediate compounds which can be more reactive, but bind more easily to non toxic, water soluble molecules in the second phase. When the reactive intermediate binds to a water soluble molecule in the liver the entire compound becomes harmless and ready for excretion by the kidneys. The liver needs certain nutrients in order to excrete these substances and send them to the kidneys. If the nutrients are not present in sufficient quantities, metabolic processes become slow and sluggish and the system back up. Once the liver creates these nonreactive water soluble compounds, these compounds can be sent to the kidneys or intestines for further breakdown and elimination. Each organ requires special nutrients to aid elimination or encourage the process of detoxification.

Understanding this process helps us look at our food as fuel to create power for our engine (our body). You would not put sugar in the gas tank of your police car, "Would You?" Your car would not run. Even beginning to think of putting as pure of fuel as possible in the engines of our bodies sheds light on the word detoxification and toxic.

Holiday Excuses

Consider the season to celebrate—Thanksgiving feasts, family get-togethers, and Christmas gifts. Traditionally it seems to have become a time for excuses, setbacks, and getting off track. Does this have to be? I think NOT.

The anticipation of the season is almost as exciting as the celebration itself. While foundations of belief behind the celebrations will vary from person to person, place to place, and country to country, the overall commonality is about gratitude for gifts. Personally, I love receiving gifts just as much as giving them. The joy that someone exudes upon the receipt of a gift is so refreshing and contagious.

Imagine at Christmas time, the eyes of a child glowing with happiness at the sight of a finely wrapped gift. The exhilaration of the child grows as he frantically tears away the ribbons and paper. The child opens a box to find a new toy or doll. Suddenly, he yells, "Thank you. This is just what I wanted." The child's smile seems to widen from ear to ear as he hugs the toy before embracing you with a huge "THANK YOU."

I realize this sight may bring back many cherished memories. However, we must transition this thought to reality. What if you were not here to relive the thought or experience this sight again this season? What if you were so sick the doctors had informed you that this would be your LAST holiday season? Let's take a fresh look at the concept of 'gift.' The greatest gift is LIFE itself. Without the gift OF life, we could have no celebrations IN life. Our life is precious and beyond descriptive value. Why is it that obesity rates are climbing drastically, sedentary lifestyles are becoming common, and we are more and more dependent upon medications to maintain our health? Sadly, we make excuses why we can't seem to find the time to care for ourselves. We have heard (or said) them all:

- I don't have time.
- I am not motivated.
- I will just fail anyway.
- It is not that important.
- I will start soon.

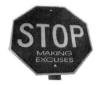

We must really understand priorities and value. Life is worth it. We must spend time involved in regular (and structured) activity as well as make more wise choices in our nutrition. It is time to rid ourselves of the excuses and begin to celebrate the greatest gift—the gift of life. In THIS season, let LIFE BE A REASON to celebrate so that your celebrations, giving, and thanksgiving may continue for years to come.

Extra Physical Wellness Nuggets

Mediocrity is Not Acceptable— Men, Where are You?

This is a recent headline from a local news website (actually my former hometown):

Tulsa made Men's Health Magazine's list of 100 worst cities for men for 2013.

One hundred cities were ranked and Tulsa made it in at #91. The magazine also gave the cities letter grades on the aspects they used to determine the rankings. Tulsa received an F for both health and fitness and a C for quality of life.

Another Oklahoma City didn't fare much better—OKC was ranked at #87.

Boise, Idaho, topped the list, while Birmingham, Alabama, came in at #100.

I must say it was a bit shocking to read such a staggering ranking regarding the men in my home state: an "F" in health and fitness? As a wellness professional, I take that personally.

Instead of complaining and doubting the veracity or validity, I wanted to offer some practical steps to make Oklahoma men climb back up on the list.

Before I begin, let's establish this premise: Men are designed to provide AND guide. This means that we, as men, are programmed to work hard, provide for our families, and live by example. Nobody would really argue the statement, "We need more male role models in society."

So here are the steps:

1. Stop making excuses. It is not OK to walk around being obese or overweight. Don't justify or rationalize your busy schedule. The longer you walk around making excuses, the more you are increasing your odds for a shorter life. You cannot work hard, provide, and be an example if you are fat, out of shape, and continue to make excuses.

2. Own your responsibility. If you have a family or children, you have an exemplary role to play. People (your family and others) watch and mimic what you do and how you do it. By not making fitness and health a part of your life, you have become a conduit for the activities of future generations (your children and your children's children).

3. Start by setting small goals. This is accomplished by setting short term goals, such as one month. If your goal is to get in shape and lose a weight; that is great.

But, SET a measurable goal (e.g. lose 8 pounds in a month). It takes a 3500 calorie deficit per week to lose one pound. This means that one pound of body fat stores about 3500 calories of energy. To lose an average of one pound per week, you must have a 3500 calorie negative calorie balance per week. This can be accomplished by eating 500 fewer calories per day, burning an extra 500 calories per day by physical activity, or by a combination of the two (recommended).

4. Clean up your nutritional habits. This can be accomplished by:
   a. Taking ½ of your restaurant order home for a future meal
   b. Don't eat while watching TV
   c. Choose lean meats
   d. Avoid fried foods
   e. Choose quality fat options (monounsaturated and polyunsaturated)
   f. Limit soft drinks

   This is not an extensive list, but this is a great start.

5. Practice the art of respect. This is done by opening the doors for ladies (chivalry is not dead unless YOU decide to kill it). Use often the words, 'Yes ma'am, no ma'am, yes sir, no ma'am, please, thank you, I'm sorry.' These words are becoming less common in our society.

When you respect others, you will begin to respect yourself enough to take care of your health.

6. Be a man. This does not mean trying to be tough, brash, and/or rude. It simply means letting your 'Yes be yes' and your 'No be no.' Too many times these days does a person's word hold NO meaning. If you are a man of your word, you will 'be a man' and become the epitome of health.

7. Don't wait on someone else to lead you. YOU make the decision today to take control of your health. It is NOT up to a pill, quick fix solution, or a silver bullet. It is up to YOU to do something about it.

Men, where are you? How does it feel to be at the bottom of the list? Remember, you are to provide AND guide. Don't point the women and children to Boise, Idaho for the example. Let them look at YOU. It will not be easy. Hard work, dedication, sweat, tears, and challenges await you. However, when you think about it, isn't that what you were designed to model? In reality, that is what health and fitness is ALL about.

Microwave Mentality

What ever happened to good old-fashioned hard, consistent work? Hasn't it always been the tried and true, sure-fire way to lasting success and results? We train and test ourselves to the max? We work for it, and we earn it. But somehow, in regard to wellness, this hard work, consistent methodology has morphed into 'I want in NOW' or what I like to describe as 'microwave mentality.' We don't want to work for it or earn it. We literally want it given to us.

As I travel throughout the world, I notice two occurrences which are becoming routine:

1. Many media-generated commercials advertising quick fix solutions to fitness—whether it be pills, exercise programs, or a combination thereof.
2. People asking me to explain the quickest way to get in shape—say in one to two months.

It saddens me to observe and hear these things. How can we undo something in 30 days (such as a poor fitness condition) that took us years to mess up—whether it is our current weight or general fitness? This is NOT reasonable or safe!!!

We need to wake up and get out of our delusional thinking! I don't mean to sound harsh. However, with the 'microwave mentality' running rampant and the obesity rate on the rise (currently 1 in 3 Americans are considered obese with an even greater percentage being overweight), allow me to ask a question…How is the 'microwave mentality' working for us (as a nation, department, or even personally)? NOT SO WELL!!!

I am often asked where I find motivation and dedication. Listen, I SEE these statistics almost daily. It is especially heartbreaking when I observe my friends and patients becoming these statistics. YES, everyone is subject to these same obesity statistics. DON'T let that be YOU! Start slow with a balanced and well thought out wellness plan. Seek the advice of a professional who has lived the life versus some media-made hyped character that you don't know. If the plan doesn't consist of both short term (1-6 weeks) and long term (3-12 months) goals, my advice is to RUN!

We look for excitement, hype, bells and whistles. I think it is high-time we stop this nonsensical thinking and get back to the basics. DON'T look for exercise plans to be fun. Rather, seek out plans that are geared toward sustained success. Fun will follow as you make tremendous personal fitness strides. DON'T look for rapid weight loss solutions. Weight loss is a symptom of behavior. Look for increasingly better choices of food/nutrition which we put in our bodies.

We spend years trying to perfect everything. Why not put this effort into our wellness? Friend, if we will begin to knit wellness into our personal fabric with a consistent, steady, and LONG TERM wellness plan, we will see our quality of life improve to new levels.

Does your thinking need an adjustment? Don't wait for a wakeup call in the form of a diseased state of wellness. Wake up NOW and DO something about it. Listen, I am not aware a safe quick fix, but I am aware (because I live it) of the results of basic and consistent hard work and commitment. Get away from the 'microwave mentality' and focus on a '4E' lifestyle change. Don't become a statistic. Become the leader you are!

Misbehavior Justification

Throughout my time of being involved in the fitness industry and in bodybuilding, I have routinely been asked the question, "Do you take steroids?" As many that have asked me that question, I am very certain there are many more who simply believe it. Since my appearances have grown and so have those who want to bring criticism (this is part of the territory), let me unequivocally set the record straight. My response to it is two-fold:

1. Thank you for the compliment!?!?!?
2. The straight-forward answer is NO!!!!!!

Though I compromised my integrity in this area many years ago, I work very hard at what I do. I spend at least 6 hours per week training with weights and at least 6 hours per week doing aerobic activity of some sort. That is 12 hours per week. I HAVE BEEN DOING THIS NATURAL FOR OVER 25 YEARS! During this time, I could probably count on one hand the times I have taken a week off. I am serious!!! It takes work!!! I travel a lot, work hard, and rest hard, but I still find the time (because I choose) to exercise and continue my regimen. My consistency, dedication, and commitment must account for something. I am grateful to God that He put that character trait in me.

Listen, I do my very best to encourage everyone in which I come into contact. I tell them there is no quick fix. You must work hard, smart, and consistently. Sadly, I see our world getting much lazier when it comes to hard work. We seem to expect things to happen without effort. I have heard it said that everyone wants to have a healthy body, but only a few are willing to pay the price.

I find myself reaching this conclusion to all those who may 'choose' to say that I cheat and take illegal drugs:

It must be their way of justifying their own misbehavior. They may think, "He cheats and that is the only way he can look like that. I am not going to take those illegal drugs." That thought has NOTHING to do with anything. It is not my fault or responsibility if others do not heed my advice and encouragement. This may seem harsh for me to say, but I ENCOURAGE those who think this of me to get your eyes off of me and get them on YOU. YOU deserve more of YOUR effort than putting that effort on criticizing me (or anyone else for that matter).

Be honest with yourself. Don't blame or justify your lack of commitment, dedication, and consistency on someone else. If you need help getting yourself going in the right direction when it comes to your internal and external health, let "Living the 4E wellness life" be your source for encouragement. I will help you every step of the way. That is why God gave the vision for this company. I want to provide motivation, information, and inspiration for you to be the BEST YOU CAN BE. Work hard, live right, and love with passion. If you follow those principles, you will find yourself encouraged and influential.

New Breakthrough

(Really?)
Lose weight and build lean muscle—WITHOUT exercise

Do you desire to return to your high school weight but hate to exercise? Do you love food and despise dieting? Do you find it difficult to stay committed? Finally—NOW—the discovery everyone has been waiting for is HERE. Now, there is something you can take that promotes targeted weight loss in the abdomen and hips, enhances the rapid development of lean muscle growth, and drastically reduces body fat—all WITHOUT having to exercise or diet.

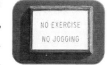

Does this sound too good to be true? It is TRUE and very REAL, and it is available to you NOW. Before I let you in on the secret, you have to promise me you will share this with everyone. I mean it! If you don't commit to share this, STOP reading now!

Are you still with me? Good! I have been exercising for over 25 years and have tried literally every diet, supplement, and workout design known to man. During my vast fitness journey and experience, and unbeknownst to my colleagues, I have been conducting experiments with dozens of people. Let me summarize just a few of the testimonials:

From: S—41 year old male

Mark, I can't believe it! I tried your discovery for only 4 weeks. In that time, my body fat decreased from 25% to 13% and my waist size went down 8 inches (from 42 to 34). I am convinced this IS the only way to go. I did not have to exercise (which I hate) and I literally ate whatever I wanted and whenever I was hungry.

From: W—34 year old female

I am amazed! I must admit I was a skeptic at first. Why wouldn't I be? You said no exercise or dieting. I am a believer now! In just 6 short weeks, I am back to my college weight and feel great. I even have my new bikini selected for the summer beach trip. Thank you!

From: Greg—53 year old male

As a professional, I didn't have time to exercise or diet. In my busy life, eating out is a way of life along with spending countless nights 'late' at the office. With what I have learned by your system

🦋 | Limitless Strength

and product, my life has changed. People ask me all the time where I train. I proudly tell them I DON'T, and then I share your secret. You have changed my life. EVERYONE needs to get on board with this TODAY. DO NOT WAIT!

Those are just three of the dozens of testimonials. Are you pumped and ready? You should be; because now you are going to get a chance to hear (for the first time) the secret behind this discovery. The product is called, NOW and FOREVER YOUNG. It is an all natural, safe and effective, dietary supplement originally discovered in a remote village of the indigenous Hawaiian people on the big island of Hawaii. During my first visit there years ago, I could not believe the way the people looked. I can admire physiques and health, but this was unbelievable. It seemed that all the women had fitness model physiques and all the men proudly displayed a lean muscular 6-pack revealing body. But how was this possible? During my time, I found no gym, plenty of fried and fatty food, and a relatively sedentary life. As it turns out–there was ONE thing they all had in common. They all ate pineapple seeds. Yes, that is right—pineapple seeds. These are not just an ordinary pineapple seeds; they are ONLY found in a grove near the village. You will understand why I cannot share the exact location. I interviewed, spent time, and began to eat them myself. I could not believe the results. I was shocked!

To wrap up the story, I decided to secure the rights to these special seeds. Now, in the form of one tiny water soluble capsule, approved by physicians, YOU can experience the same effects as the indigenous Hawaiians in the village AND my test group. Supplies are limited as I am currently on backlog with orders. However, I am offering this special deal to my friends first. Contact me through email for YOUR 6 month supply of this amazing product. At $89.93, it is literally a give-away. However, my friends are 'everything to me.' No exercising, no dieting, ONLY that lean look for YOU. Get it today while supplies last.

God bless you in your pursuit of health.

New Breakthrough Part Two: Scams, Shams, and Quackery

(A MUST READ follow-up)
Lose weight and build lean muscle—WITHOUT exercise

Let me begin by stating I put out the previous section as a short article on social media. This was a social experiment of sorts. My intent was to leave it visible for at least 72 hours to observe response. Additionally, everything in the previous section introducing the new breakthrough supplement was **untrue**. However, everything was perfectly legal. In researching supplement advertising, I was shocked at how much was indeed OK to say. Basically, the ONLY thing the FDA will not allow is something along the lines of "…treats,

❧ | Limitless Strength

cures, or prevents disease or illness." All else seems to be fair game.

To make matters worse, there is SO much of this out there that people generally don't know how to tell a fake or fraud. Here is a non-exhaustive checklist of scam, sham, or quackery alerts:

1. If it sounds too good to be true, it is.
2. If it says 'all-natural', that doesn't mean it is safe. Some poisons are 'all-natural.'
3. If it promotes the sense of loss (e.g. get it NOW, supplies are limited), stay away!
4. If is asserts a physician's blessing, ask yourself the identity and field of study of the so-called physician. Then, check him/her out thoroughly.
5. Testimonials mean nothing. Anyone can lie.
6. Eating fattening food and living a sedentary life will increase your chances of illness and pre-mature death.
7. Having a healthy body and mind ALWAYS requires hard work, dedication, and commitment to a lifestyle. NOTHING of real value comes easy.

Finally, even though most of my readers know me well, I was totally blown away by the response. In just over 48 hours, I had totaled over $3000 in orders. I could have taken the money and shipped seeds. Sadly, most 'pineapple seeds' are so small they are barely visible AND probably, nobody would have really questioned what they would have put in their body anyway.

As a wellness professional, I endorse quality products that I use myself. In this day and age, it is sad to say that this 'scam' sold more 'seeds' in 48 hours than I could sell legitimate supplements in a 48 days.

Lastly, this experiment was NOT designed to make anyone feel foolish. It was designed to educate and inform. I trust everyone learned a few things. Please, work hard daily on your total wellness. We ONLY get one body and one mind. **Treat them with extreme care and caution.**

Where to Eat Out and What to Order!

Being a person who really goes to the extreme in nutrition, I sometimes get asked questions that include the following:

- What do you eat when you go out?
- Do you ever cheat on your diet?
- Where do you go when you eat out?

Believe it or not, I do eat out at times. I always try to select the best option. I choose to not 'cheat' as I have a completely different picture of that principle than you have probably ever heard which I will explain in further detail in moment. However, the questions above can best be answered by outlining a few principles that anyone can follow, anytime:

> ❦ | Limitless Strength

1. Avoid the free bread and chips. If you must have one piece of bread or a handful of chips, take them and politely ask the server to take the rest away. These two are major culprits to the obesity problem because of their high glycemic properties. Basically, they promote a high insulin spike which signals our bodies to store fat. This does not take into consideration the very poor nutritional properties of these two foods.

2. Choose a reasonable portion of lean protein. This can be in the 6 to 11 oz. size in the baked or grilled variety. Some examples include: tilapia, salmon, chicken breast, lean steak, and bison.

3. Choose a mixed green salad with the dressing on the side. This is far superior to a simple iceberg lettuce bowl. Obviously, the best dressing, if any, would be a simple vinegar and oil. However, if that does not suit your taste, DO NOT put the dressing on that salad. Put the tongs of your fork in the dressing before putting the tongs into the bed of greens. This will cut down sharply on the amount to dressing used.

4. Choose grilled or steamed vegetables with the butter on the side. The same principle applies to the butter as the dressing if you must have the buttery taste.

5. Avoid baked or mashed potatoes and instead select sweet potatoes or red skin potatoes. The white potatoes are extremely high on the glycemic index and the others mentioned are only moderately glycemic.

6. Drink plenty of water with your meal. This will promote a full feeling and curb overeating.

7. Chew your food slowly until it gets soupy in your mouth. This helps wonderfully with the digestive process. Further, it takes the stomach 20 minutes to connect with your brain to tell you that you are FULL. This makes it imperative to slow down when eating.

8. Avoid the dessert. It is normally loaded with sugar and certainly high glycemic.

9. Avoid all fried foods. These are simply unhealthy... enough said.

Now to address my concept of 'cheat' meals: If I realize these cheat meals promote storage of fat and deterioration of my health, why would I choose to PUNISH myself in that manner? It is the equivalent of making A's all week then going to the Principal's office on Friday to ask for a spanking with the largest paddle he can locate!

Notice I did not name specific places or restaurants in which to eat. One can incorporate these simple principles relatively anywhere. Print these and try them out. Before long they will become second nature to you and generate a second wind to your life and health.

❦ | Limitless Strength

What Everybody Ought to Know About Overeating

I saw two neighboring restaurants recently which had signs reading "ALL YOU CAN EAT." Obviously, for those of you who know me quite well, I have not visited either place. My non-visitation, however, is not based on the taste or quality of the food. It is based upon another, often confused and misunderstood, concept altogether. What is this concept? It is the concept of *gluttony*, also known as overeating.

Before you stop reading and possibly get defensive, I ask that you allow your mind to see a different perspective. Gluttony is the insatiable appetite for something that will never bring fullness of satisfaction, which is a much deeper definition than the often repeated (and shorter) definition— that of "eating too much."

8 Reasons to Avoid Overeating

1. Your stomach can only hold so much. It can stretch of course, but the digestion process is very poor because of the enormous amount of food.
2. During the eating process, there is an immediate sense of gratification or happiness. However, it is followed by an even longer sense of remorse and generally poor feeling.

Mark Sherwood, ND |

3. The stomach is made a certain size for a reason. With too much food to process as energy, the reserve energy is in turn stored as fat.

4. Eating too much promotes obesity, which can in turn lead to heart problems, diabetes, high blood pressure, and joint pain. Obesity is epidemic in our world.

5. The propensity to eat too much can become habitual in nature making you a slave to food. Most have no idea how many calories they eat.

6. Food addiction is harder to break than addiction to alcohol and drugs. This is based on the fact that we must eat to survive.

7. Gluttony can make you forget that having *enough* food is a blessing. We live in a land of plenty rather than a land of not enough.

8. Food is designed to give the body a source of sustenance and energy rather than a pleasurable experience. That is why a key food measurement is the 'calorie'—a unit of ENERGY. The pleasure of the experience is sharing a meal with loved ones.

I ask you then—is the practice of gluttony beneficial? I will be bold in my own assessment. I fear we have fallen prey to having it too good for too long. We may have become spoiled to the core in expecting to always have *more than enough*. Abundant food, in my opinion, is both a blessing and a curse. We are blessed to have it in abundance, but at the same time

❦ | Limitless Strength

our abundance has given us a sense of entitlement. We have eating contests and claim the contestants are athletes while at the same time realizing eating too much is damaging to our bodies. We want to *save room* for more when we really are gathering more than we can ever utilize. Many of our days' schedules are made based on *when we will eat*. We joke and laugh about eating too much like it is a badge of honor.

Maybe, just maybe, we don't want to admit we have become prisoners of our abundance! All you *can* eat should rather be viewed as all you *should* eat. My friend, I ask you to really think about this! Reassessing the concept of gluttony can literally save your life.

Is Cardiovascular Disease (CVD) Preventable?

You make the call!

This is a loaded question indeed. Is the number one cause of death for men and women in the U.S. preventable? On the surface, one would quickly assume, "no."

Upon close inspection of the heart attack numbers, I began to ask myself some very hard questions:

Are they preventable? How can one train in a prehabilitative manner? Do our actions really make a difference?

To answer these questions, let me present some facts. The majority of all cardiovascular disease deaths (51%) are because of coronary artery disease (CAD). Hear t attacks, resulting from CAD, cause about 425,000 deaths in the U.S. annually. About 35% of all heart attacks are fatal. There are 8 major risk factors for CAD (I am only briefly summarizing each):

1. Abnormal Blood Cholesterol
   a. Without getting too technical, generally speaking, a goal of total cholesterol 200 or less is desirable, 200-239 is borderline high, while 240 or greater is high.
   b. You want your LDL (bad cholesterol) to be below 100 and your HDL (good cholesterol) to be at least between 40-59, while being over 60 is better.
2. Hypertension (High Blood Pressure)
   a. 120/80 on average is normal
   b. 120-139/80-89 prehypertension
   c. 140-159/90-99 stage 1 hypertension (Medical Urgency)
   d. 160+/100+ stage 2 hypertension (Medical Emergency)
3. Tobacco use (enough said)
4. Pre-diabetes
   a. Normal fasting blood glucose levels are 70-99 mg/dl.
   b. Fasting blood glucose level between 100-125 mg/dl on two separate occasions is called pre-diabetes.
5. Family history

> a. If you have a male blood relative with a history of CAD prior to age 55 or a female blood relative with the same events prior to age 65, you may have a genetic link to CAD.

6. Sedentary lifestyle
   a. Lack of participation in at least 30 minutes of moderate intensity physical activity on at least three days per week, for at least three months.
7. Obesity
   a. Waist to hip ratio greater than 1.0 in males and >0.8 in females
   b. Percent body fat >20% in Men and >28% in women
8. Age
   a. Males age 45 or older and female age 55 or older

Now that I have laid out these 8, let's examine the irrefutable remedies of each:

1. Cholesterol
   a. Increase physical activity
   b. Better nutritional choices
   c. Decrease body fat
   d. Better manage stress
   e. Control diabetes
   f. Stop using tobacco products
2. Hypertension
   a. Same remedies as cholesterol

Mark Sherwood, ND | ❦

3. Tobacco use
   a. Really? Do we need a remedy here?
4. Pre-diabetes
   a. Increase physical activity
   b. Better nutritional choices
   c. Decrease body fat
5. Family history
   a. Can't change this one. I bet some of us wish we could.
6. Sedentary lifestyle
   a. Increase physical activity
   b. Better nutritional choices
   c. Decrease body fat
   d. Better manage stress
7. Obesity
   a. Increase physical activity
   b. Better nutritional choices
   c. Decrease body fat
   d. Better manage stress
8. Age
   a. I can't help here either!

Of the 8 major risk factors, WE have DIRECT CONTROL OVER 6! You cannot convince me or anyone else using logic that many instances of CAD are not preventable. I have said many time that ***WELLNESS*** IS A RESPONSIBILY. We should live that way!

Lastly, heart attack deaths are a cumulative result. Behaviors over time add up to a lethal consequence. We must stop the tide and reverse the trend.

So, as this section is partially entitled, "YOU MAKE THE CALL", ask yourself this question—Is cardiovascular disease preventable with YOU (your capacity to modify your risk)? If the answer is YES, NOW is the time to take a serious look at our lives and avoid becoming an unnecessary statistic!

PART 2

Emotional Wellness

Always fun?

Many times in my travels, I have heard people say, "I just hate exercising; it is no fun!" In short, what they may be saying is, "I won't exercise because it is no fun." The lack of fun has become the excuse. Exercise doesn't have to be torture all the time; sometimes it can indeed be fun. But, not ALL the time! However, whether it is 'fun' or not should not be the determining factor in deciding to do something that has proven beneficial toward the length and quality of life. Let's compare exercising to work. Is it always 'fun' to go to work? Either way, a person still must work to get paid (at least I do). I hope you certainly do 'love' your job each day. But, even if you didn't 'love' it, would you simply stop going?

Allow me to bare my soul a moment in regard to the 'fun' element of exercising. Some days it is drudgery!! I don't feel like doing it! It is not 'fun' all the time!

Philosophically, I am thinking it is really not supposed to 'fun' either. Exercise, like life, is full of challenges and places of resistance. We are continually encouraged and motivated to face life's challenges head on. We hear all the inspirational speeches. When we meet a challenge head on, oftentimes we discover a new level of depth in our character—we mature and grow. Folks, exercise is NO different. Face this challenge head on! It is NOT

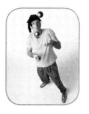

supposed to be always 'fun.' However, I am fully convinced that the fruits of your labor in fighting the 'no-fun exercise excuse' will produce both internal and external benefits in not only your physical health but in every area of your life.

This challenge is NOT TOO BIG for you! It is just what life ordered!

7 Lessons I Learned that Lead to Complete Freedom

The definition of ignorance is having no knowledge of a matter in which you must decide, deliberate, or act. On the contrary, stupidity is having intimate knowledge of a matter in which you must decide, deliberate, or act, *then* acting opposite the knowledge in a way which brings contrary and sometimes dangerous actions to oneself.

So, with the establishment of two definitions, we can now discover how to be free from both. It begins with gathering knowledge. The knowledge to any subject is available by activity seeking out the correct source. Always seek information based on experience and science. When information is gained, you therefore avoid the label of being 'ignorant.' With the lack of ignorance, however, we now gain *responsibility*. Yes, we are now responsible for our actions. Inside the concept of responsibility lies the ability to avoid being 'stupid.'

❦ | Limitless Strength

With the remedy to avoid being stupid or ignorant clearly defined, let me pass on some incredible knowledge designed to bring real change to your life.

7 Lessons that Lead to Freedom

1. Eating too much sugar leads to obesity, inflammation, metabolic syndrome, diabetes, and heart problems, among others. We can avoid eating too much sugar by utilizing the glycemic index food chart in regard to our carbohydrate intake.

2. Our water intake should be at least 1/2 our lean body weight in ounces. This is very important for hydration and detoxification.

3. Lack of regular exercise (defined by the American Heart Association as at least 3 times weekly for 3 months) can lead to a sedentary lifestyle, weight gain, and obesity.

4. Spending more than you make and living outside your means leads to debt. Debt is like wearing handcuffs and it will steal your freedom. You DO NOT have to keep up with the Jones'. Just be YOU and you will experience freedom.

5. Do not try to change others. You can't do this anyway. Trying to 'make' someone change is futile and will zap your emotion, energy, and time.

6. Avoid needless conflict. This simply means minding your own business. If you don't like something, leave the situation if possible. If it is not possible to leave immediately, stand by your principles in regard to your life.
7. Keep a close reign on your mouth. Words can bring destruction or construction. If you don't have something good to say, don't say it. Don't miss a great opportunity to shut up. Words spoken rashly will always return with vengeance. A kind word can subdue even the greatest anger.

Putting this knowledge in it's correct place in your life (your mind and heart) is critical to allowing the knowledge to become firmly rooted. Once there, you have the opportunity to experience great growth and freedom by 'being neither ignorant or stupid.' The correct use of this knowledge lends itself to something called wisdom. With wisdom comes health, wealth, and freedom. As the 4E philosophy goes, you will be well physically, emotionally, intellectually, and spiritually.

Generational Wellness

As I travel around the world, I have become somewhat of a people watcher. Obviously my passion for physical wellness and my compassion for those who struggle with weight issues has become a part of the lens through which I often view

❦ | Limitless Strength

people. Though my book is intended to reach the masses, this section is specifically geared towards parents and those who wish to be someday.

Let me begin by describing a heartbreaking scene. I am sitting in an LAX terminal as I observe a father and mother walking towards me accompanied by their children. I estimate the parents' age to be in their 40s with their two girls' ages to be in their 20s. They all were visibly showing discomfort as they walked. Additionally, all four were at least 150 pounds overweight. The daughters were even larger than their mother. I must admit a deep sense of sadness I felt as I thought about what I was really seeing. It was much more than just a severely obese family. It was a family that undoubtedly will have to deal with the enhanced risk of disease and death at a much earlier age than should be expected. I thought about these daughters one day having children. I even wondered what others may be thinking. Do we really treat 'those people' different? Will they have to purchase two seats on the airplane? I thought about when/how this generational pattern of 'un-wellness' began. When will it end? Will it ever?

Let's face some statistical truths. Today, nearly 4 in 10 Americans are obese. Predictions are dire with the obesity rate rising in teens and preteens. Someone has to step up and break the cycle of generational 'un-wellness.' Parents (and those who wish to be), YOU ARE THE ONES called to step up and break this dangerous cycle. Do something now in regard to changing your life, extending the quantity of your life, enhancing the quality of your life, and starting a generation-changing pattern of wellness. Here are some things you can begin right now:

- Get a medical check-up
- Start a walking program
- Gradually change your nutritional habits by adding more natural foods and vegetables
- Drink more water making it your main liquid intake
- Seek the advice/services of a trusted wellness professional who lives out what he/she teaches
- Don't take shortcuts or fall for quick fix gimmicks

This subject, I realize, can be very personal and very emotional. However, when we are speaking about generations, we are speaking about a very real subject that affects OUR REAL FUTURE.

Please take these few words seriously and pass them on to those you know who need to hear this. It is coming from someone who really cares. This may be uncomfortable and toe-crunching to talk about, but it is badly needed across our world. This is not an advertisement for my services, but because of my passion, I will help as a trusted wellness professional. I threw that our there to eliminate an excuse (e.g. no person cares or is willing to help) people often use. Friends, excuses will get us nowhere. This time, this day, this hour is the time for parents (and those who wish to be) to stop making excuses and passing the buck. I challenge you to make the commitment to be THE ONE to begin a pattern of generational wellness in your family.

How Do You Find Peace in the Midst of Chaos?

This is a question I have asked myself many times over the years. As a single father, life has been anything but a piece of cake. I receive responses regarding my presentations, sermons, tweets, and blogs that seem to hold the theme that I, Mark Sherwood, seem to have it ALL together and have no problems in which to handle. Do you really believe that? I certainly hope not!

Listen, I have to get up each day and face issues like everyone else. Though you may or may not know my entire story (you will soon enough), trust me when I tell you that I have had many extremely difficult and painful occurrences come my way. Just to get a brief glance into "my world of issues," you must realize that being the sole provider for three children for over 11 years is less than the "ideal" situation. However, things happen in life, and we are forced to play the cards we are dealt. So what exactly is it about myself that allows me to press onward and upward? It is something I have honestly and earnestly explored. The basis of my exploration has been based on what I see occurring in the world today.

More and more people are discouraged, beat down, depressed, and in a really bad state of mind. Statistics do not lie as the pharmaceutical industry has blossomed with the introduction and inclusion of anti-depressant drugs. With the economy in decline and the family unit being torn apart at alarming rates, is it any wonder people feel less than positive?

So here is my answer to what sets me apart and drives me on: I put attention and effort to all areas of my total person (intellectual, spiritual, emotional, and physical), and I seem to notice that I try a little bit harder than most.

Intellectually—you must NEVER stop learning. Find something to read or a class to attend. Stimulate your mind.

Spiritually—cultivate your relationship with a higher power. I focus mine on my relationship with God.

Emotionally—put yourself in situations, activities, or hobbies that produce peace and calm in your emotions.

Physically—this is the piece that is normally ignored and left off. It takes effort, planning, prioritizing, and discipline. Our bodies were made to be active and NOT sedentary. Activity (in the form of exercise movement) actually brings about a state of peace in our emotions. When our emotions are at peace, we all tend to function more effectively spiritually and intellectually.

Friends, I put a lot of attention and effort into all FOUR areas of my being. THAT is how I find peace in the middle of chaos. I owe it to myself and to you to take care of me. I want you to be encouraged, uplifted, and dream big. I believe in YOU.

Hyper-vigilance
(and the physical results of an over-stimulated life)

We all know what it is to be "over stressed." Though we may not be able to really understand it physiologically, we KNOW when we have arrived at that state. Additionally regarding today's world, there is little doubt we all understand the necessity of staying alert and even somewhat hyper-vigilant. The bottom line—you must stay 'on your toes' at all times. During these times, there is a powerful biological response occurring inside our bodies. This response is called a sympathetic nervous system arousal (SNS–often called the 'flight or fight' response), which is quite necessary for our survival. During this response, we see a substantial production of cortisol, which in turn stimulates the production of glucose which must be managed by the hormone insulin.

Herein lies a major problem in law enforcement. We begin to live in a state of chronic stress without much thought to long term effects. Basically, it becomes a 'normal' part of life and we FORGET how to relax.

So what is cortisol and what does it do?

Cortisol is a hormone produced as a by-product of cholesterol. It is one of the primary stress hormones that is secreted from the adrenal glands.. It is necessary to maintain normal internal (heart rate, blood pressure, digestion, blood sugar balance and even the sleep wake cycle) balance and function during times of great and negative stress, including positive stresses such as exercise and a hard but satisfying day at work. We forget that positive stress can also be taxing on our system. Without cortisol, the body would be unable to respond to stress.

Our bodies produce cortisol to manage stress, but when stress is present constantly, cortisol production rages out of control until the adrenal glands no longer can keep up the work. Cortisol has the same long-term side effects on obesity and diabetes by dysregulating insulin and blood sugar metabolism. This is one way the 'insulin animal' is set in motion. Not getting enough sleep is as bad as being a 'sugar-aholic' or a couch potato. A stressed system leads to an insulin resistant system which lends itself to metabolic syndrome and the onset of obesity with the change in body composition. No one wants to be "FAT".

Elevated cortisol resulting from chronic stress can lend the following conditions:

- Obesity: Elevation of body fat, particularly visceral or abdominal fat. This type of fat poses a huge risk to the cardiovascular system. An increase waist to hip ratio > 1 in. men and > 0.8 in. women equals high risk for heart disease, myocardial infarction (heart attack), high cholesterol levels and hypertension.
- Memory loss or impairment
- Decrease in lean body mass- sarcopenic obesity. As stated above, the term is a mix of two different words-

| Limitless Strength

Sarcopenia and Obesity. "Sarcopenia" meaning loss of muscle and "Obesity" which is the increase in fat percentage as described in Medical text.

- Decrease in bone density
- Increase in anxiety
- Increase in depression
- Mood swings
- Decreased sexual drive and desire for intimacy
- Alteration in the hypothalamic pituitary end organ axis. This can result in negative changes in menstruation, menopausal, and andropausal (male menopause) symptoms.
- Decrease in the immune response and increase in susceptibility to infection
- Elevation in blood pressure

From where does cortisol come?

The body naturally produces cortisol, which is considered one of the stress hormones alongside norepinephrine and epinephrine. There are certain signals that trigger the hypothalamus' secretion of a hormone called corticotrophin releasing hormone or CRH. Stress is one of these signals. CRH travels to the pituitary gland, one of the master glands, and causes secretion of ACTH into the blood. ACTH travels through the blood stream to the adrenal glands, which sit on top of the kidneys, and stimulates the release of CORTISOL. This hormone cascade happens on a rhythmic cycle in the body. However, chronic stress is constantly stimulating this cascade to produce cortisol, never allowing blood/serum levels to return to normal. Constant and continuous elevation of cortisol lead to the adverse effects mentioned above. All of the body systems suffer and the immune system is seriously diminished.

The overarching action of cortisol in times of stress is to reduce all other metabolic activity not directly involved in fueling the high energy demand that is necessary to address the stress. This task is accomplished by enhancing the production of the high energy fuel glucose (blood sugar) via regulation of protein, carbohydrate, lipid and nucleic acid metabolism. Cortisol raises the blood glucose (blood sugar) levels by antagonizing the secretion and actions of insulin to inhibit peripheral glucose uptake, which tells the liver to make more sugar. Yes, this in turn can literally stop body's ability to utilize fat as fuel.

The actions of cortisol on protein metabolism are mainly catabolic (breaks down good quality muscle tissue). Cortisol causes an increase in protein breakdown and nitrogen excretion, lending a negative nitrogen balance. If the body is in a state of negative nitrogen, it is metabolizing its own muscle as fuel. The action of cortisol causes a mobilization of amino acid precursors from tissues such as bone, muscle, and connective tissue due to protein breakdown and inhibition of protein synthesis and amino acid uptake.

It promotes little argument when I state we live in a fast-paced, microwave world. Everything and everyone moves fast. We must have it NOW. It is good to know that elevated glucocorticoids (adrenal hormones) protect us under stress. However, as stated above, the over production of such hormones long-term can lead to immune dysfunction, loss of muscle tissue, skeletal bone loss and thinning of the skin. In conditions of their deficiency, such stresses (chronic) may cause low blood pressure, blood sugar imbalances, metabolic syndrome, Diabetes, Obesity, and even death.

All that said, we could be 'doing' all or most of the 'right' things (exercise, training, and nutrition) but still experiencing debilitative results in our health.

Here are several techniques for law enforcement to combat a hyper-vigilant lifestyle:

1. Maintain and foster friendships outside of law enforcement.
2. Develop hobbies outside of law enforcement skills.
3. Take regular vacations with your family (I recommend one every two months for at least 2-3 days).
4. Practice quiet introspective time at least 10 minutes daily (this can mean prayer, meditation, or simply just silence).
5. Understand you CANNOT change the world (or your community) alone. Keep things in perspective and just do YOUR PART.

6. Be willing to seek and receive counsel from ministers, license professional counselors, or colleagues.
7. Be HONEST WITH YOURSELF in regard to your own hyper-vigilant state as it relates to your health.
8. Re-learn the skill of relaxation—take a break from the world, work, computers, and cell phones. This can be hard but very freeing.

Let's not let the hyper-vigilant life kill us from the inside out. Be committed to doing something about it starting today.

Slow Down and Get Real

Everything is so fast paced these days! Fast food, fast cars, fast service, faster speeds, etc. When does it end? I honestly don't think it will ever end. Is it any wonder the world is literally overrun with anxiety? Even in my area of expertise, fitness and health, I can see the effects our ultra fast society. As you are at the check-out station at the grocery store, you can see advertisements on magazines featuring such topics as…"Lose two dress sizes in 7 days"…"Drop 30 pounds in thirty days"…"Get your beach body in 3 weeks without exercise."These are just a few. Are you kidding me? We are all reasonable people. Does this sound credible? How about too good to be true?

In reality, I wish it were that easy. I have been exercising for over 25 years on a consistent basis. During some of my best years, I put on a whopping 6-7 pounds of muscle. Yes, that is what I said! I only added 6-7 pounds of muscle in a good year! That doesn't seem like much, but if I only added 5 pounds of muscle a year *for ten years*, guess what? I will have added a *massive 50 pounds of muscle*. This is body transformation at its best.

Listen folks! Life is a marathon, not a sprint. The healthy and smart way to positively change the composition of your body is **NOT** found in fast, fad-like remedies. It **IS** found in good old-fashioned, consistent, well-planned exercise and dietary principles. We should realistically only lose 2-4 pounds per week. Planning with the *marathon mentality* will tremendously help you in your drive to achieve better health.

Managing Personal Risk

We all understand the concept of 'risk.' Risks are something we take daily. They can be in the form of driving to work, walking across a street, or perhaps risking a dollar on a slot machine. We are basically speaking of 'probability management' or 'managing the odds.' If we really think about it, life is much about probability management.

This concept applies beautifully to our overall wellness. Examples:

- If we eat sensibly and correctly, we lower the 'probability' of acquiring diabetes before we are 70.
- If we exercise regularly, we decrease our 'risk' of having cardiovascular disease.
- If we maintain our physical conditioning, we lower the 'odds' of losing our temper prematurely.
- If we work on staying in proper posture while standing and sitting, we lower the 'probability' of having back troubles.
- If we get proper rest, we decrease our 'risk' of becoming fatigued.
- If we stop texting or using a phone while driving, we decrease the 'odds' of causing a traffic collision.
- If we behave recklessly in the area of nutrition, choose to be sedentary, are not paying full attention to our actions, or are not getting enough rest, we increase the 'probability' of premature death.

You get the idea. It is ALL about the probabilities. Using the above examples, here are a few tips to more effectively manage your personal risk:

1. Eat sensibly. Every meal counts.
2. Exercise regularly. Perform cardiovascular activity 5-6 days per week (as easy as a 30 minute walk) and strength training 2 days per week.

❧ | Limitless Strength

3. Maintain a proper balance between work, family, rest, and play.
4. Give full attention to driving. Do not text or talk on the phone while you drive.
5. Select proper relationships. Avoid becoming overly invested in one-sided relationships that drain and never fill up.
6. Practice good sleep hygiene. Try to get at least 8 hours per night.
7. Pursue education. Keep reading and learning to stimulate the brain throughout your life.

So there you have it. Consider carefully the probabilities as you utilize your daily allotment of 1440 minutes.

The Exercise—Sanity Connection

Has someone ever told you to "go take a walk and cool off"? Hopefully you experienced the benefits of listening to that advice. It is very helpful to understand why these benefits appear.

When our emotions are heightened by anxiety, frustration, anger, or fear, it seems as if our minds go on 'lock-down mode' where we can't think and process information as easily as we can when we are calm. Realize this is normal as our body/mind has transitioned to the 'fight or flight' mode. Your primal design is forcing you to decide whether to run for your life or to fight for your life.

These are bodily reactions that are natural and reasonable. However, to live in this state constantly would no doubt have catastrophic physical and mental health effects. It would literally push our sanity meter to the max.

The sure-fire way to combat this high intensity, mind clogging, and sanity testing occurrence is exercise. Yes, even a simple walk will do. When you do take that walk to 'cool off,' chemicals are produced in your brain that will metabolize the chemicals that were produced to cause the 'fight or flight mentality.' Therefore, there is a calming of your emotions, a decrease of your intensity, an unclogging of your mind, and a return to a sense of sanity.

In today's world, economic uncertainty and unpredictability is the norm. With this sort of norm, it is no wonder some people have become stressed to the max to feel as if sanity is a long-past state of mind. This is why exercise MUST become a part of everyone's lifestyle. It is NOT an option anymore. IT IS A MATTER OF SANITY.

We DON'T Have to Accept Failure or Mediocrity

Have you ever heard it said, "It is not IF but WHEN?" These words feed the 'no option' mentality. I have heard this statement applied to getting sick, gaining extra fat pounds, and going in debt, among others. Tell me—is it a 'rule' that we have to get sick, gain extra fat pounds, or get in debt? I fully realize it is 'accepted' and even 'expected.' However, 'why' does it HAVE to be?

The answer lies in the very DNA we have created. This DNA is not biological; it is psychological. Many have talked themselves into believing lies. Friend, just because someone believes something, does NOT mean it is true. For centuries, people 'believed' the earth was flat. Only when sailors sailed and did not 'fall off the edge' did we find out different. Clear your mind with me a minute and explore some new possibilities. Let's examine the possibility that we CAN be relatively free of illness, relatively free of excess fat pounds, and relatively debt free. Do those conditions seem appealing? Do they give you a sense of wonder, awe, and peace? If the answer is YES, then let's further explore what we can do to make these conditions a reality.

How to live relatively free of illness:

- Eat a healthy diet of lean meat, vegetables, and fruit.
- Drink plenty of water—at least ½ your bodyweight in ounces daily.
- Get plenty of rest—at least 8 hours per night.
- Maintain a regular exercise regimen—workout with weights at least twice and perform at least 150 minutes of cardiovascular activity weekly.
- Maintain a healthy balance of emotions—not over-reacting to uncontrollable life events.

- Continue the pursuit of learning—never falling into the trap of thinking there is no more you can learn.

How to relatively free of gaining excess fat pounds:

- Same as above

How to live relatively debt free:

- Don't spend more than you make—live within your means.
- Work hard and stay committed.
- Give a percentage of your income to charity.
- Save for your future or emergencies.
- Pay yourself a percentage of your income for enjoyment/entertainment/travel.

As you can see, the answers seem simple. It is up to us now what we will do. We DO NOT have to accept failure or mediocrity. Friend, let's live by a new set of truths—truths that provide benefit and future. Let's stop believing lies and start LIVING with possibility!

Don't Miss the Moments

Recently while on a business getaway with my wife, I was struck by the beauty of the surroundings...mountains, waterfalls, and sunshine along with that indescribable sound

❦ | Limitless Strength

of joy. At that moment, it occurred to both of us that we had been to many such places throughout our lives. Unfortunately, even though I had been to many beautiful and enchanted places in this world, I had not really 'been there' at all. I had forgotten to embrace the beauty and majesty of the moment and location. Even though I was fully engrossed in the magnitude of this particular moment, I felt an overwhelming sadness that I had missed many others.

You probably know exactly to what I am referring…You are in a location that you should be totally taking in, but because of the hustle and bustle of the world, you are not really 'there' at all. Physically you are there of course, but are your there emotionally, intellectually, and spiritually? It is funny how that lines up with the 4E philosophy–learning how to experience peace through the daily renewal of the physical, emotional, intellectual, and spiritual person. Certainly, we ALL have a need to experience this fullness of life, what I call THE WELLNESS LIFE. With that said, I am bound and determined to not 'miss the moments' and make sure I am totally 'there' when I am THERE.

To ensure that no longer happens to me (or any of my friends like YOU), I have developed a 3-prong exercise guaranteed to make you 'experience the fullness of the moment.' Here it is:

Step 1: Ask yourself the question, "Where am I?". The answer may seem obvious at first, but I want you to go a bit deeper. Don't just name the location; describe it. If you have to do this out loud, so be it. Where are you, what does it look like, what does it smell like, etc.

Step 2: Ask yourself the question, "What am I doing?". I am not just referring to 'right NOW', I am talking about what you are doing in this place. What brought you here, what have you done while you are here, and what are you planning on doing. You get the idea.

Step 3: Ask yourself the question, "How do I feel?". This is where I want you to really dig deep. What emotions do you experience: joy, happiness, peace, etc. If you are feeling happy, say "I am happy." If you are feeling peace, say "I am so at peace."

By conducting these 3 simple steps, you will not 'miss it'. We all are so very blessed with so many good things and opportunities. I sincerely believe, however, that we often miss the blessing (or greatly shortchange it) because we fail to 'inventory' the moment. It is much like taking a 4D picture with your entire system utilizing your physical, emotional, intellectual, and spiritual senses. My friend, enjoy the moments. Experience them in 4D! Don't miss any of them and totally embrace the moment of NOW.

Extra Emotional Wellness Nuggets

The Daily One-Minute Exercise That Will Change Your Life

1 440 minutes—our total time allotment every day. How we 'spend' our time is indicative of our priorities. Whether we spend or invest our time derives our level of return. If we spend our minutes wisely, we attain a great return and vice versa. Following is one tip regarding one minute that will change your life immensely.

Spend at least one minute every day in total silence.

This will require some work, but I guarantee you the payout is enormous. Silence is something we seriously lack in this crazy, hellish-paced world. In preparation of your silent minute, you must eliminate all noise except natural noise (wind, air, rain, etc.). This means getting away from the cell phones, computers, music, TV, and people. Once in your quiet place (whether outside or inside), you may either use a stop watch or wrist watch to time your silent minute. Just relax, take a deep breath, and let the silence begin.

During the silence, you may experience a bit of anxiety at first, but trust me, it will quickly pass as the sweet moment of peace from chaos will envelope you. I practice this routinely and have realized that the more I do it, the more I crave it. Yes, I said CRAVE IT. We were designed for rest (even as God did and directed). However, we must re-learn this gift of silence.

Employ this tip starting today. It only takes a minute!

Diaphragmatic Breathing

A Relaxation Technique to Lower Stress

We all know what it feels like when the Sympathetic Nervous System (fight or flight) is aroused—increase in blood pressure, heart rate, respiration, adrenaline, muscle tension, and perspiration. We sometimes "try" to calm down, but find ourselves in much the same mental position.

Diaphragmatic breathing is a sure-fire method to quickly bring some calm to the situation. Basically, this type of breathing can force a Parasympathetic Nervous System

❦ | Limitless Strength

(relaxation) arousal—a decrease in blood pressure, heart rate, respiration, adrenaline, muscle tension, and perspiration. This probably sounds too simple and good to be true, right?

Here is how it is done (try it right now):

1. Lie flat on your back with your hands resting on your abdomen (near your naval).
2. As you inhale, force your abdomen to push upward.
3. As you exhale, move your abdomen back downward.
4. When you begin to get a rhythm with this, put a little resistance (with your hands) against your abdomen as your push it up and then back down during the breaths. **Do this for at least 1 minute.**

Follow these steps, and you will force a Parasympathetic arousal, guaranteed! Use this method regularly in times of great anxiety or when having difficultly falling asleep. You will learn to enjoy this as much as I do.

PART 3

Intellectual Wellness

Are You Aiming at the Right Target?

In my roles as a wellness practitioner, motivator, and educator, I am constantly harping on my patients, clients and listeners to set clear, reasonable, and attainable goals. Goal setting is extremely important as it provides a roadmap for success. Clear, reasonable, and attainable goals are set in time increments—one month, three months, six months, etc. Reaching these micro-goals along the path to your macro-goal ensures you are on the correct course. I cannot underestimate the importance of goal setting as it provides clear targets in which to aim or focus. But what if one were to aim at an incorrect goal because of misinformation or lack of knowledge? Can you imagine what one would think upon arrival at an incorrect goal? There would be no satisfaction and no joy—only sadness and disappointment.

Goals are important in life as well. It is critical we have both micro and macro goals whether they be family, employment, relational, or financial. These goals should be set based on as much information as one can uncover. They should be well-formed and well thought out.

Unfortunately, I have discovered a truth about many of today's more common goals. You see, I have pursued incorrect goals and upon arrival, found myself completely disappointed. This article would spill into a novel should I begin to spell out each of my missteps. Many today set their goals based on finances (or 'treasures' as my favorite book utilizes) and/or the attainment of success. Allow me to point out definitions of each.

Treasure—A quantity of precious metals, gems, or other valuable objects.

Success—1. The accomplishment of an aim or purpose. 2. The attainment of popularity or profit.

When we put much of our life's effort into attaining these 'goals', we will become sadly disillusioned. Neither will bring fulfillment and happiness. Many say that money can make one complete. However, more money will only make you more of what you already are.

So what is a correct goal? What is the target in which we should aim?

I learned the answer from a child. You see, I spoke at a school about a year ago. There was another event held later that day in which I spoke as well. The young lady was present at both. To cut to the chase and abbreviate the story, the young lady saw me at another recent event. I must admit I didn't recognize her (I speak to a LOT of people). But, WOW, she knew me. In the midst of the crowd, she approached, hugged me, looked me in the eyes, and said, "Thank you." She went on to tell me I gave her hope and encouragement. I saw a gleam in her eyes that I will never forget. Being an emotional guy, I began to cry. The look in her eyes communicated clearly the answer we all need regarding goals and targets.

At THAT MOMENT, it hit me right in the heart. The CORRECT goal is to pursue giving others hope and encouragement. When one strives to achieve that goal, the real 'treasures' will pile up and 'success' is experienced in the most profitable way.

To give hope and encouragement is to build an overflowing treasury and a legacy of success.

Friend, BE ENCOURAGED TODAY AND HANG ON TO HOPE!

Commitment Phobia

Phobia is defined as an extreme or irrational fear of or aversion to something. When I mention this condition, we often link it with the fear of crowds, the fear of heights, or the fear of being closed in. However, I want us to examine the epidemic condition of commitment phobia. It has permeated our society to the point we fail to acknowledge its existence. The belief that we are 'entitled' to certain things has fueled the spread of commitment phobia. In all truth, we are entitled to nothing except the choice of how hard we want to work for those things/people we deem most important.

Commitment phobia begins with the following (faulty) beliefs:

1. I deserve this or that…
2. I shouldn't have to work that hard…
3. There has got to be a shortcut…
4. I don't need to work, God will supply all I need…

5. People owe me…
6. I am entitled to this because I am an American…

When these ideas become part of our normal speech, they quickly become our internalized beliefs. They guide our lives and shape our destinies. Friend, this deceived belief system forms the basis for the development of commitment phobia. Has your belief system become distorted and confused? Do you suffer from commitment phobia? To determine if you have commitment phobia, ask and answer the following questions:

1. Do I fear commitment because of fear of failure?
2. Do I have a generally negative belief system when it comes to goal setting? Do I think I will fail?
3. Do I resent those who seem to frequently achieve goals and embrace challenges?
4. Do I have a negative view of myself (e.g. I am a failure)?

If you answered 'yes' to any of these questions, consider yourself commitment phobic.

There is, however, good news. Here are some small things you can do (I call it my commitment phobia vaccine) to overcome and eliminate this condition forever (I encourage you to post these in the areas you most frequent):

1. Give yourself permission to fail. Nobody is perfect. You will fail from time to time. It is a fact of life.

Limitless Strength

2. Learn to forgive yourself. As stated in #1, you will fail. Be just as quick to forgive and cut yourself a break.
3. NOTHING comes without hard work and commitment. Great things require great effort. Great effort is rewarded with great achievement. Stay the course.
4. Nobody (including you) is designed to be a failure. You are designed for great things. There is only ONE you. You are unique and special.
5. It is not how many times you fall that matters; it is how many times you get up. The mark of a champion is found in rising up when others count you out.

Let's make commitment phobia a permanently exterminated condition, and that starts with YOU! Put this proactive and positive commitment phobia vaccine in your heart, mind, vision, and words today.

Consequences—Fact or Fiction?

I have had the pleasure of speaking all around the world to students and adults about the power of consequence. I do my best to inform all about our freedom of choice. What an amazing freedom that is! However, each choice has an attached consequence, whether good or bad.

As I have spoken on the topic, it has become very clear to me that if the consequence does not quickly manifest, the power of the choice tends to diminish. Let me give you this example:

I have three wonderful children whom I love dearly. Because of my love, I want each to excel as a human being and be happy in all their years on the earth. When they made great choices (they make plenty by the way), I tried to reaffirm the power of their great choice very quickly by acknowledging my pride in them. This was my way of giving them a good consequence in response to a good choice. As we all know, these affirmations must be done in close time proximity to the original choice to maximize their effectiveness.

One the flip side, if one of my children made a bad choice (we ALL do), I did my best to quickly affirm a consequence (if not already experienced by them) that the original choice was not optimum. We like to call this 'discipline'. We don't like the word in this context, but we all understand its necessity. As with good choices/good consequences, these disciplinary actions must take place as close to the choice to maintain efficacy.

If these consequences had NOT followed closely or at all to the choice, would the desired or undesirable behavior have been repeated? I think your answer would be much like mine and look something like: "I HIGHLY DOUBT IT!"

As I transfer this logic to wellness, I will paint a picture for you:

Imagine a steamy donut or piece pie! Think of a large enchilada with loads of rich creamy cheese! How about a large bucket of corn chips with queso and salsa in which to "load up"?

What do you see? What do you think about? Do you see a consequence on the horizon if you indulge?

Everything in moderation is OK of course. However, if the consequence of our overindulgence in these types of unhealthy foods does not appear quickly, we oftentimes continue the behavior. Guess what? The consequences only likely show up in a minimal way…we may experience indigestion or a slight stomach ache followed by a sugar-crashing nap. The real consequences appear 5-10-20 years later through a buildup of plague which result in a stroke, obesity with its own list of attached ailments, or outright death.

What do I see when I think of those food items described, you ask? I see a grenade set to explode in your stomach, a vial of cyanide in a time-release capsule, and slow-working acid set on eating every organ in your body without your knowledge.

I know that sounds severe, but if it does get your attention regarding the GUARANTEE of consequential results whether now or later, then my mission is successful. Friend, take a long thoughtful look at your choices along WITH consequences!

Do You Have a Plan?

Before you build something, you must have a plan. No person that I know starts construction on a house without first developing, examining, and approving a plan. How foolish would it be to start construction and have little or no idea where to begin, where to continue, or where to begin?

Unfortunately, in the world of fitness, I see this "lack of planning" as the norm rather than the exception. The reason for this is actually very simple...We don't understand the extreme importance of the plan. Just like house plans, there are many fitness/exercise plans. When choosing a plan, there are some basic foundational principles in which the plan must adhere.

1. Is it balanced—trains all parts of the body equally.
2. It incorporates weight training—utilizing progressive resistance techniques.
3. It incorporates cardiovascular training—aerobic training at least 4-6 times a week for at least 20 minutes a session.
4. It includes short terms as well as long term goals—plan is designed for lifelong "marathon mentality" participation rather than the "quick fix mentality."
5. It is success driven and designed—successes are obtained with relative ease rather than focusing on failure (e.g. training to failure).

If the plan does not adhere to these basic principles, my advice is to scrap it and keep looking.

❦ | Limitless Strength

You must have a plan designed for success in building your fitness level. Choose wisely, follow the plan, train with purpose, and enjoy lifetime fitness and success. Be 4 ever fit!

New Year's STOPS

At each year end and New Year beginning, we hear talk of resolutions, new starts, and better habits. Many of these are geared towards our desire for better health. There are many great ideas regarding resolutions, and equally great ways of making them reality. We can, however, be so focused on the 'start' that we forget what we need to 'stop.' In this section, I thought I would address a few things that we need to STOP doing when we make 'new years' resolutions.'

1. STOP setting your goals too high (e.g. I am going to lose 30 pounds 1 month).
2. STOP attempting to make drastic changes in your diet (e.g. I will never eat a cookie again).
3. STOP trying to radically change habits (e.g. you haven't been to the gym at all, but now you promise to go 5 times a week).
4. STOP being so hard on yourself (e.g. if you fall off the wagon one day, forget it and move forward).
5. STOP trying to be like others (e.g. you are unique. No person is like you).

6. STOP making excuses (e.g. you control what you do with your time).
7. STOP blaming your failure on others (e.g. my workout partner did not show up).
8. STOP trying to find motivation through others (e.g. I have to have someone make me do it).
9. STOP telling others what you are going to do (e.g. let your action speak. If you don't accomplish what you say, you set your own self up for failure).
10. STOP having a failure mentality (e.g. telling yourself you will never be able to do this).

Puts these 'stops' into your new year's resolutions. By doing this, I believe you will see more success in your 'starts.' Make each year, the greatest year, of your life. STOP doing the things that hurt YOU and do not promote YOUR success.

7 Ways to Avoid Surgery— Saving You Boatloads of Cash

Information that is not valued has no lasting value. I make that statement with emphasis. People spend hard-earned money to seek advice and information from experienced professionals and practitioners, such as myself. When I am questioned about cost, I embrace the opportunity to educate regarding

❧ | Limitless Strength

the concept of investing in your health. With that said, lets take a look at the cost of some common surgical procedures.

Average Cost of Common Surgical Procedures

- Heart Surgery **$100,000**
- Gastric Bypass **$22,000**
- Liposuction **$3,000**
- Knee Replacement **$50,000**

It is astounding to see these numbers, but the doctors who perform these procedures certainly must have the required expertise. They don't, and should not, work for free. Oftentimes this is not all 'out-of-pocket', as we depend on our insurance to cover an amount or percentage. If one does have a procedure as described above, what do you think would happen to your monthly insurance premium? Yes, you guessed it; it is destined to increase over time.

What if I told you there are several less expensive things you could do right now to greatly increase your chances of avoiding these procedures all together? Would that interest you? If so, keep reading…

There is little debate that these procedures are often needed because of a poor nutritional, highly stressed, and sedentary lifestyle. Here is a list (with potential costs) of what you can do NOW to regain or maintain your health.

7 Ways to Regain & Maintain Your Health

1. Utilize quality protein drinks in the morning.

   I recommend 20-25 grams of powdered protein mixed with 12-14 ounces of unsweetened almond or coconut milk. This highly dense morning protein meal starts the day off by regulating blood sugar. Remember, how you start often sets the tone for how you finish. Cost of quality whey protein: $50-$80 for 2 pounds. This results in an average cost of this meal being between $2-$3. This sure beats an egg, cheese, and sausage muffin at your favorite fast food establish in both price and quality.

2. Walk a little each day.

   This sounds almost too good to be true, but walking is the best form of exercise. Obviously, I recommend progressing to jogging if possible and including weight training (at least 2 days weekly). This helps keep the extra weight off, assists with circulation, and helps with detoxification (through sweat). *The cost on this is FREE.*

3. Eat a salad for lunch with a 5-6 ounces of lean protein.

   At a restaurant, you will pay between $8-$12 for this. At home, however, the price will be as little as $4-$5.

4. Practice the diaphragmatic breathing technique to relax.

❦ | Limitless Strength

This helps big time in the area of stress (your response to outside stimuli). *The cost on this is FREE.* Discover the diaphragmatic breathing technique in which I discussed earlier.

5. Do not eat carbohydrates after 7:00 p.m.

This will keep insulin down, assist with sleep, and aid fat metabolism while you sleep. *The cost on this is FREE.* You may even consider it a gain as it saves the expense of that late night pastry or bowl of ice cream.

6. Eat whole and real foods as much as possible.

Sounds simple enough, but it may require a redesign of your grocery shopping plan. Buying whole and real food can increase your normal grocery budget at first by 20-30%. However, after a time, you and your family will begin to eat less as the food becomes more nutritious.

7. Apply this advice with the proper value it holds.

I normally require a nearly $100 hourly fee. Because I care for each of you, I am giving you this advice for FREE without having to make an appointment. If the last two statements sound arrogant, that is not my intention. I simply desire that you view the information as very important and highly valuable.

There you have it! Following these 7 rules will decrease your chances of having to have the procedures above performed on you. So which costs more? What is the better investment?

I urge you to invest now as to NOT PAY later. I desire for you to have a higher quantity and higher quality of life.

Talk it—Walk it—Live it

I have been asked many times, "Mark, how do you consistently maintain a wellness program?" Those who question sometimes add, "You have been able to keep it going for over 25 years." Without thinking too much, I normally answer, "I just make it a priority." With further thought regarding my *normal* answer, I want to share some deeper insights into why **maintaining a wellness program HAS TO BE a priority**. It is important to establish that by *wellness program*, I am referring to a consistent exercise routine, an awareness of what and how many foods I eat, and a working knowledge and application of the supplements that I utilize.

As a representative and ambassador for both internal and external wellness, I have learned one thing…**I have to talk it, walk it, and live it**. I cannot say one thing and do the other. You see…there are far too many people in this world that simply talk a good game. I want to paint my life canvas as being the real deal. **If we really do want to accurately represent a pathway to wellness, we must become persons who have actually travelled our own personal pathways and subsequently talk from experience**.

Here is a blunt example:

❦ | Limitless Strength

Why would I listen to someone about exercise, wellness, or nutritional supplementation, when it is apparent by looking at and spending time with them, they are **NOT** living it out. I am not being judgmental in this; I am stating the obvious. If a person has a wellness 'how-to book' in one hand and a cigarette in the other, what kind of message does that send? If a person takes two multi-vitamin caplets and chases them down with a shot of whiskey, what message does that portray?

We must truly examine and be brutally honest with our own internal motivations and fears, and then learn to listen and be vulnerable to our own consciences. When we live in a way which is contrary to what we want, we cannot make excuses. Each of us has responsibility for our own life, and we hold the keys to their own level of external and internal wellness.

Why is maintaining a wellness program a priority in my life?

- I want to enjoy an enhanced quality and quantity of life.
- I want to get the most out of each day.
- I want to be as illness and disease free as possible.
- I want to have a healthy mind and body.

Does this list contain traits or characteristics of what you want out of life? If so, it is time to start letting your words match your actions, and in turn, direct your life. All I am saying is this…words can be cheap. **Don't just talk it! Walk it and live it!**

Re-evaluating Value

When we speak of value, we normally think of dollars and cents. How much does it cost? How much is it worth? It this (or that) a good value (monetarily)? We even place value on 'time' when we say, "Time is money." You get the idea!

However, I want us to take just a moment to reflect on what 'value' really means. Basically, 'value' is set by how important and/or precious we believe or perceive regarding a person, place, or thing. Many 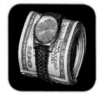 times, these perceptions align themselves with the perceptions of others who have similar assessments.

Ok, now let's take it one step further and attempt to add some 'sense' to the 'dollars and cents.' How much is TIME really worth? Is there a dollar amount as it pertains to seconds, minutes, hours, days, etc.? I am specifically speaking about your life 'time' on Earth. I hope that provokes more in-depth thoughts regarding 'value.' Your life 'time' is valuable. It is actually priceless because you cannot buy it back. So let's RE-EVALUATE VALUE. If we 'value' time the way we say we value time, let's put real effort into making our life 'time' longer and of higher quality.

As we all know, there is basically one area of our life (that we control) that affects the quality and quantity of life. That one are is our choices and decisions regarding our activity and nutrition. Statistics have shown that inactivity and poor nutrition are lessening both the quality and quality of our lives. There is little (if any) argument to these statistics. Maybe it is time we take a step back and gain a fresh perspective as to how we 'value' our life 'time.' It is TIME to place OUR EFFORT where it belongs. Take the step (literally) toward more daily activity and making better choices with nutrition. RE-EVALUATE VALUE as it pertains to your life 'time.' Both you and your life 'time' are worth it.

Extra Intellectual Wellness Nuggets

Pre-habilitate Your life

Pre-habilitation is a form of strength training designed to prevent injuries BEFORE they occur. However, this term can be effectively used in your personal life, business, and employment. Under this context, let me define pre-habilitation this way: "It is the management style of incorporating proactive and preventative measures or actions designed to prevent mistakes, delays, deficiencies, and the development of unwanted business culture BEFORE they occur."–Mark

I will spend the next few sections literally 'hammering' this point home. If heeded, YOUR life will be permanently altered for the better.

As we examine the elements of this management style, we see application for our daily lives. Let me begin by asking you a couple of questions:

- If you could prevent having the intense pressures of out-of-control debt, would you do it?
- If you could avoid the pain of a broken close personal relationship, would that appeal to you?
- If you could escape the experience of having excessive amounts of fatty tissue on your body which caused serious health issues and pushed you into trying nearly anything for a 'quick fix', would that interest you?

Hopefully, the answer to each of these questions is a resounding YES!

The solution, to preventing, avoiding, and escaping the aforementioned conditions, lies foundationally in the concept of pre-habilitation. Now is the time to pre-habilitate our lives! We may not be able to avoid the 'current', but we can pre-habilitate our future to a great extent. Let's 'pre-habilitate' questions 1-3 in order:

- Pre-habilitation of out-of-control debt begins with the formation of a budget. If you are not familiar on 'how to do it', ask a close personal friend or financial advisor for help. Find someone to hold you accountable to living within your means. Sell unnecessary luxury items to eradicate debt and build

♟ | Limitless Strength

an emergency fund. I subscribe to the Dave Ramsey school of thought on this issue.

- Pre-habilitation of close personal relationships begins with not letting everyone into your close personal circle of life too fast. Too fast and too soon normally results in disaster. Let the relationships develop with time. In time, the relationships will grow or dissolve naturally. Maintain a very small (2-5) group of very close friends. They should be people who are not afraid to tell you when you are wrong and are bold enough to appropriately praise you at the same time.
- Pre-habilitation of your health begins with scheduling daily appointments with yourself for activity, which is outside of your normal employment duties. This will provide great benefit because a body that is not moving is either dead or rapidly on the way. We don't need to speed up this process on our own by not being active. Make wiser choices nutritionally. Reduce saturated fat (and increase good fats) and processed foods, and increase the intake of fruits, vegetables, and lean proteins.

Pre-habilitation as a management style in business or employment is excellent as well, but can also be used very effectively in our personal lives.

Pre-habilitate Your Family

This is the second in a series of five on the subject of pre-habilitating your life. As you recall, the last section centered on pre-habilitating our personal lives. This one focuses on pre-habilitating our families.

One more time…

As a reminder, pre-habilitation is a form of strength training designed to prevent injuries BEFORE they occur. However, this term can be effectively used in your personal life, family, business, employment, and church. Pre-habilitation defined: "It is the management style of incorporating proactive and preventative measures or actions designed to prevent mistakes, delays, deficiencies, and the development of unwanted business culture BEFORE they occur."–Mark

As we examine the elements of this style as it applies to our families, let's begin, as usual, by asking a few questions:

- If you could prevent having the horrible disappointment of communication problems with your spouse or significant other that resulted in over-the-top misunderstanding, would that appeal to you?
- If you could avoid the pain of hearing shocking information about your child's unexpectedly negligent or bad behavior, would you do it?
- If you could escape the trauma of experiencing divorce, would that interest you?

❦ | Limitless Strength

Hopefully, the answer to each of these questions is a resounding YES!

The solution, to preventing, avoiding, and escaping the aforementioned conditions, lies foundationally in the concept of pre-habilitation. Now is the time to pre-habilitate our families! We may not be able to avoid the 'current', but we can pre-habilitate our future to a great extent. Let's 'pre-habilitate' questions 1-3 in order:

- Pre-habilitation of communication problems begins with setting aside a time to simply 'talk and listen.' Schedule a mutually convenient time with your spouse or significant other to discuss the day. This can be done in the evening before bed. I recommend allotting 10 minutes each to talk. During the 10 minutes, the other person is only to listen. This can be a time to discuss highlights, issues, needs for clarification, or expressions of gratitude. Make the ground rules clear, and make sure each person understands those rules. This is a time that must be carefully guarded. It is an appointment that must not be canceled absent exigent circumstances.

- Pre-habilitation of being surprised about disparaging information about your child in similar to how you would handle communication with your spouse. This however, is a totally different level. I recommend scheduling a daily family dinner time. This is a time in which the TV is off, dinner is on the table, and the family is enjoying a meal together. Each child is given the opportunity to share the events of their day—highlights, problems, struggles as well as issues with friends, teachers, and yes—parents. There should be no interruptions when the child speaks. However, a clear time limit must be held as other children need time as well. The parents can manage this effectively. If there are serious issues that need to be discussed in private, make time and opportunity for that to occur at the first available moment.

- Pre-habilitation against divorce occurs at the outset of any pre-marriage relationship. Marriage is not like testing a car. It is serious business with amazing results from success and disastrous heartaches from failure. I recommend dating someone for at least 2 years. This may seem strange, but time will prevail in uncovering weaknesses and vulnerabilities. In accepting and loving these weaknesses and vulnerabilities, a deep love relationship can be forged. There should be common interests and parallel beliefs regarding faith. Having opposing faiths can drive a nearly insurmountable wedge. I also recommend a stringent counseling process, especially if this is the first marriage.

There you have it. We have utilized pre-habilitation as a management style in our family to prevent some of the most dreaded consequences.

Pre-habilitate Your Employment

This is the third in a series of five on the subject of pre-habilitating your life. As you recall, the last article centered on pre-habilitating our families. This one focuses on pre-habilitating our jobs.

As we examine the elements of this style as it applies to our employment, let's begin, as usual, by asking a few questions:

- If you could prevent having a difficult working relationship with a co-worker, would that appeal to you?
- If you could avoid the challenge of a less than desirable relationship with a boss, would you do it?
- If you could escape the drama of gossip affecting your job, would that interest you?

Hopefully, the answer to each of these questions is a resounding YES!

The solution, to preventing, avoiding, and escaping the aforementioned conditions, lies foundationally in the concept of pre-habilitation. Now is the time to pre-habilitate our jobs! We may not be able to avoid the 'current', but we can pre-habilitate our future to a great extent. Let's 'pre-habilitate' questions 1-3 in order:

- Pre-habilitation of working relationships begins with healthy boundaries. Healthy boundaries are marked and defined early on. If the boundaries have been muddied and are unclear, it is more difficult (but NOT impossible), to re-establish. Healthy boundaries mean not sharing too much personal information with co-workers. Keep it mostly (if not all) business. Try to avoid visible emotional swings that promote your own loose lips. If a co-worker wants to talk personal, it is polite to listen but with limits. Remember this is your job. If you are not a licensed professional counselor, don't try to solve the problem. Listen, don't say too much, and when their talking is concluded, politely excuse yourself from the conversation and get back to work. Limit getting too close to one person. Be equally friendly to all in your immediate environment, but do your best to keep your words few and your work plentiful.

- Pre-habilitation of a less than desirable employer-employee relationship begins with hard and consistent work. Arrive at work ON TIME. At least 15 minutes early is on time. There is nothing more a boss dislikes than a chronically late employee. It sets the tone for an entire organization. If you want to have 'boss

❦ | Limitless Strength

problems,' just make it a practice to be consistently late. Another pre-habilitation concept is to NOT leave early. If you get paid for 8 hours, work 8 hours. This is reasonable and expected. This should not be something you are made to do rather something you choose to do because of your integrity. Don't over extend lunch breaks. In other words, simply be ON TIME all the time. And lastly, don't share your opinions with the boss or others unless specifically asked. If the boss wants your opinion, let him/her ask for it. Let your work product do the talking.

- Pre-habilitation against gossip on the job is the easiest and most difficult at the same time. We all have a tendency to share information. The bottom line is this: If you don't have something good to say about someone, don't say it. When idle and unsubstantiated chatter begins, the story changes. It can destroy lives, reputations, and your employment. Get the facts before you speak. If the facts are not your business, stay OUT of it. If you do find out something that is a negative about someone, keep it to yourself. If the person in whom you are speaking is not present, the conversation does not need to take place. If it does, excuse yourself and choose to not be a part. Obviously the only caveat to this would be an internal, supervisory-directed investigation into a matter. A common sense approach applies in this area as well as the golden rule: do unto others as you would have them do unto you.

There you have it. We have utilized pre-habilitation as a management style in our employment to prevent some of the most dreaded consequences.

Pre-habilitate Your Business

This is the fourth in a series of five on the subject of pre-habilitating your life. As you recall, the last article centered on pre-habilitating your employment. This one focuses on pre-habilitating your business.

It is a common goal or dream of many to progress professionally into a management position or individually to business ownership. To that end, let's examine the elements of pre-habilitation as it applies to your business by asking a few thought-invoking questions:

- If you could prevent having a 'communication gap' between management and your first-line supervisors, would that appeal to you?
- If you could avoid fairly constant employee turnover and build great loyalty, would you do it?
- If you could reduce employee sick time and lower worker's compensation claims, would that interest you?

❧ | Limitless Strength

Hopefully, the answer to each of these questions is a resounding YES!

The solution to preventing, avoiding, and escaping the aforementioned conditions, lies foundationally in the concept of pre-habilitation. Let's pre-habilitate your business! We may not be able to avoid the 'current', but we can pre-habilitate our future to a great extent. Let's 'pre-habilitate' questions 1-3 in order:

- Pre-habilitating a potential 'communication gap' is fairly easy. It starts with communication. Communication should take place not only through inter-department memos and emails, but through person to person communication. Hold bi-weekly team meetings at a pre-determined time. Have a clear-cut agenda and do not 'chase rabbit trails.' The meetings should focus on information, job-well-done reports, and complaints. Every person should be given the opportunity to speak. Any questions about management decisions should be answered by the team leader. If an answer is not available, the team leader should have the answer for the next meeting. Open and regularly scheduled person to person communication is the key to pre-habilitating the 'communication gap.'
- Pre-habilitating employee turnover and disloyalty is found in the process of value and consistency. People

want to be valued and appreciated. At the same time, people want to know what to expect. The best way to drive people away from an organization and foster an environment of distrust is to never acknowledge people as people. Employers should make it a habit to frequently visit the workplace. Talk with your employees and ask about their families. If someone in your business does an excellent job, quickly and publicly praise them. Praise the behavior that you want repeated. On the other side of the coin, if someone really messes something up, act quickly, decisively and consistently. Don't give your employees reason to claim unfairness or unequal treatment.

- Pre-habilitating use of sick time and worker's compensation claims can be accomplishment with a company-wide wellness culture. This is a culture practiced and established by leadership. A wellness plan will be far less effective if not top-down AND bottom-up driven. The plan should be voluntary and participatory-based. Families and dependants should be included. The workplace should be 'illness-proofed.' Avoid bringing donuts and cakes to meetings. Make walking and activity normal business practices. Let the employees see you, the boss, being publicly active. Remember, if you lead your business in wellness, your employees will follow. Over time, it is agreed that increased activity and better nutrition improves wellness.

❦ | Limitless Strength

There you have it. We have utilized pre-habilitation as a management style in your business to prevent some of the most dreaded consequences.

Pre-habilitate Your Church or Ministry

This is the fifth in a series of five on the subject of pre-habilitating your life. As you may recall, the last article centered on pre-habilitating your business. This one focuses on pre-habilitating your church or ministry. Even though the implication may be for only ministry leaders or pastors, there are many applicable principles for your individual ministry (i.e. your actual life).

In case I have not made my point and to ensure we maintain our foundation, pre-habilitation is a form of strength training designed to prevent injuries BEFORE they occur. However, this term can be effectively used in your personal life, family, employment, business, and church. Pre-habilitation defined: "It is the management style of incorporating proactive and preventative measures or actions designed to prevent mistakes, delays, deficiencies, and the development of unwanted business culture BEFORE they occur."—Mark

Those of us involved in ministry, whether full-time or part-time, want our ministries to be both exemplary and effective. We must balance the following discussion with this disclaimer…People will get mad, and it is impossible to please everybody. To that end, let's examine the elements of pre-habilitation as it applies to your church or ministry by asking a few thought-invoking questions:

- If you could prevent some of the church/ministry splits that happen so frequently in America's church, would that appeal to you?
- If you could promote an environment of consistency and integrity in your church/ministry, would you do it?
- If you could reduce staff turnover and promote staff loyalty, would that interest you?

I know the answer to each of these questions is a resounding YES!

The solution to preventing, avoiding, and escaping the aforementioned conditions, lies foundationally in the concept of pre-habilitation. Let's pre-habilitate your church/ministry! We may not be able to avoid the 'current', but we can pre-habilitate our future to a great extent. Let's 'pre-habilitate' questions 1-3 in order:

- Pre-habilitating the frequent church splits can be a bit complicated. The complicated segment is dealing with the complexity of people. The answer, however, is found in two basic principles: A. Don't spend too much time dealing with disgruntled people. People will get mad—it is just the nature of ministry. You will have opposition. However, it you spend too much

❦ | Limitless Strength

time trying to convince the disgruntled few, you will lose the content and happy majority. B. If people want to leave, LET THEM LEAVE. They most likely left some other place to grace you with their presence. Be nice, polite, consistent, and loving, but AT THE SAME TIME, let them leave if they choose.

- Pre-habilitating a consistent and integral environment begins with practicing that in your own area of greatest influence. Teach people what to expect in your home and inner circles by modeling consistency and predictability. Don't be scattered and lack schedule. If you do, it will invariably show up very pronounced in your public ministry. Return phone calls and emails in a timely manner. If you blow people off by using the old "I am too busy in ministry" excuse, you will lose people. Listen, ministry is about example more than words. If you are too busy to get back with someone in 48 hours, have someone (maybe an administrative assistant) touch base with those trying to reach you. Believe me, this practice alone will pay huge dividends towards forming a strong foundational and consistent environment.

- Pre-habilitating staff turnover and promoting staff loyalty is very similar to number 1 and 2 (directly above). However, just realize you are MUCH closer to this group (meaning they know YOU better and that makes you much more vulnerable). Protect integrity with this group. DO NOT act flaky with them. Promote and acknowledge often the behavior you want repeated. Be consistent with your expectations. If they begin to act disgruntled, confront it with love immediately. Don't let it sit and fester because it will spread. If a staff member wants to leave, help them leave. That's right, help them leave! Maybe God is calling them elsewhere. Allow God to have His way as you lead your staff.

Obviously, there is MUCH more in this area we could cover. Perhaps, I will address it again soon.

There you have it. We have utilized pre-habilitation as a management style in your church/ministry to prevent some of the most dreaded consequences.

PART 4

Spiritual Wellness

Things Have NOT Been Easy

(A look INTO my life)

Because my whole life centers around total wellness, and the fact that I realize people form opinions based on first impressions, I thought I would dispel a few things about my own life. Things have NOT been easy for me. On the contrary, I have had many hard times. Allow me to bare my soul a few moments. I believe it is extremely important because I want you to share a glimpse inside my heart.

When people notice my stature and physique then hear my enthusiasm, passion, and abilities when I speak, I realize some may see a person who they believe has not had too many struggles. Let me begin by painting you a picture of a somewhat pudgy teenager with little to no muscle tone who was bullied. I clearly remember being much weaker and smaller than most and some of the 'cool' kids actually hitting me on the head and flipping my somewhat large ears. I was the subject of some ridicule but never allowed anyone to see my hurt. Being nice and friendly to all was my coping mechanism. My relationships with girls were nonexistent. Though I was a 'nice' guy, I really did not have the exterior looks to appeal to the 'cute' girls in my school. But, I did have some girls want to 'just be friends.' I was fairly gifted athletically and used sports as my 'escape' too. As I write this, I suspect some memories may be rekindled in your life.

After being fairly successful in baseball, I was able to play baseball on a very partial scholarship at a small NAIA school. Because my social confidence was somewhat scarred, I put ALL my effort into the athletic arena and was able to work my way to nearly a full scholarship by my senior year. After college, my dream of playing major league baseball was never realized, although I was able to play briefly as a bullpen catcher at the AA level here in the States then a year in the South Australian Baseball League.

While in Australia, something very strange happened to me. I had a lot of spare time during the day and decided to try lifting weights. This experience drastically changed my life. After I returned to the US, two things happened: 1. I joined the police department, and 2. my body (and the way people viewed me) apparently had changed. Now, all the girls wanted to date me and be 'more than friends.' Because I had literally NO experience in this area, I made horrible choices regarding the women in my life. I have been married and divorced twice since but did have three wonderful children. Make no mistake; divorce has a terrible affect on kids. In both marriages, I made mistakes of course, and suffered though false allegations. Some false allegations resulted in me being publicly humiliated. In these days of the internet, things can get posted and mysteriously become the Gospel. One of my favorite sayings is 'trying to undo a rumor is like trying to un-ring a bell.' It simply cannot be done. It truly seems to be the norm these days to believe the juicy rumor without testing its veracity.

If that wasn't bad enough, my mother suffered from depression and a somewhat tumultuous relationship. This ended unexpectedly when she took her own life some 10 years ago. My heart breaks anew each time I speak of this event. I simply miss her so much. Since I am an only child, much of this burden still rests heavily on my shoulders. My father, who is still alive, has not been the same since and has been a much different guy.

In addition to these struggles, I was a single parent for quite some time. Trying to raise children in this world with no family to assist was difficult.

I am just touching on some major struggles I have had without going into great detail. I do not say all this to make you say 'poor baby.' After surviving and continuing to fight, I hold my head high with enthusiasm and passion. You see; I know what it is to hurt and suffer loss. The scars I have will never go away; they are deep inside my heart. Because I have the benefit of looking 'back' on those aforementioned struggles, my compassion for others is unexplainable. I deeply care! I love my father, my children, and all people in a manner that seems unfathomable to me. Only God has made this possible. It is NOT about me being religious. Religion makes me want to vomit. It is, however, about my real relationship with God.

Things have not been easy for me. So the next time you see or hear me, realize there is depth in my experience and sincerity in my passion. Please forgive me if you feel I have been too forthright, but you need to know that things (and people) are not always what you see on the surface.

God bless you.

A New Kind of Detoxification

I hear the word detoxification used many times when it comes to our physical health. I am totally in to that type of thing, knowing that ridding our bodies of the junk (or toxins) can only enhance our health. I would suggest everyone explore this type of detoxification often (at least one every couple of months). Hey, it can only help, right? However, I want us to take a much broader view of detoxification in the following paragraphs—a detoxification that not only includes food, but much more.

Let's consider a detoxification of the following: food, information, habits, and people.

1. Food—It is extremely beneficial to go on all natural cleanse. There are many on the market today, but I recommend simply doing this for a period of 7 days:
   a. Drink only water
   b. Eat only real plant food (fruits and veggies) at least 4 times a day

| Limitless Strength

   c. Consume no fried foods

   d. Eat only quality (baked or grilled) portions of fish and chicken and other meats

2. Information—there is a ton of toxic information out there. This information is radical in nature and forces the belief that you can achieve 'unbelievable' reductions in weight in a rapid amount of time. This should be done gradually over time (maybe 1-2 pounds per week). This should not be done by drastically reducing your daily caloric intake (forcing a starvation mode), but should be done through portion selection and control along with daily activity. Hard and consistent work is the key. Lifestyle change is the ultimate goal. Avoid the 'quick fix' information. After all, how can you fix something in 30 days that has taken you years to mess up?

3. Habits—daily habits are the key. It is really about placing time into your priorities. For example, you get 1440 minutes per day. Where do you spend it? Is activity (exercise) important? If so, manage your time correctly. Schedule activity into your schedule as you would make an appointment with yourself. There is no need to feel guilty. You are valuable, and the better you value yourself, the more you will value others.

4. People—some people can suck the very life out of you. You KNOW who they are. Learn to say NO. By not saying NO, your response to them (stress level) will

become increasingly hostile. This promotes negativity in your mental health and enable them to continue 'leaching' behavior.' This will not only do you good but will serve them well. Toxic people can be destructive just as the toxins in unhealthy food.

I recommend taking a weekly inventory using the above-criteria regarding your need for a good detoxification. This type of broad-reaching detoxification will provide beneficial results in not only your physical health but your emotional, intellectual, and spiritual health as well.

The Sacrificial Cost of Freedom

Delays in airports are often boring and unwelcome. However, during a recent such experience, I was convinced this particular delay was divine in nature.

In my eye and earshot, I watch a young father (approx. 35) and his young son (approx. 8) listen as an older gentleman shared his life of sacrifice. You see, this conversation began with the father and son approaching the older gentleman (wearing a Vietnam veteran hat) and requesting the man recount his military experience. I could honestly see this father seizing the opportunity to teach his son the ultimate meaning of life.

I listen intently as the man shares about bloodshed, fear, war, friendship, and loss. I see his eyes as he speaks. They clearly show his visual recollection of the painful events. After a few stories, I am engrossed further as the young boy asked the older gentleman, "Was it worth it?" I felt myself literally hold my breath as I waited for the answer. After what seemed like minutes (it was probably only a few seconds actually), the gentleman answered, "Yes, I would do it all again."

I watched as the young boy paused, moved forward, hugged the older gentleman and said, "Thank you!" The father then shook the gentleman's hand before walking away with his arm around his son.

I stayed close and continued to listen as the gentleman's wife tells her husband, "I am so touched by that. If only people understand how good God is to us." She continues, "If only more fathers would be like that…"

Tears began to well up in my eyes as I ponder in my heart what just occurred. You see, I really believe our current generation lacks in knowledge of sacrifice. We all have freedom to speak our mind and live our lives because of sacrifice. Sacrifice has alway been synonymous with bloodshed (i.e. someone has to die and pay with their life). There is a cost for freedom. Oh, if we would all stop and ponder the sacrificial cost for freedom. FREEDOM IS NOT AND NEVER WILL BE FREE!

For the young boy (as well as myself), I am certain this 'life lesson' is one that will never be forgotten. Also, in this case, I am thankful for delays. From the bottom of my heart–to all those who sacrificed for my freedom, I say, "THANK YOU!"

How does this apply to us, you may ask? It applies very appropriately. EVERYTHING in life requires hard work and sacrifice. When those are appropriated, good things happen and freedom from something (addiction, bad behavior or habits) results.

Those Eyes

It is said that the eyes are the window to the soul–a glimpse into the very heart of the real person. 18000 miles and an entire continent away I looked into the eyes of thousands of children in Africa. During my fairly constant speaking engagements and strength presentations on other continents (especially Africa), I have been blessed to speak to thousands of people. However, I did not see what I expected. My expectations were, I must admit, to see eyes hungry for something quite different than I was accustomed to giving. My preconceived ideas formed the opinion that I would learn of a culture much different than my own–a culture lacking proper nutrition, adequate shelter, or clean water. Though these conditions were readily apparent at times, what I saw in those eyes was eerily familiar to a picture I have seen steadily for the past 10 years plus. For in those eyes, I saw the hunger for role models of hope–real heroes that stand up, stand out, and speak up for values, ethics, morals, and truth. It seems as I ponder further over my experience, I am more convinced than ever that people's real universal need is hope, faith, and belief to be able to achieve something better in life–to reach for and attain a goal or dream despite their current circumstances.

When hope is demonstrated and communicated, circumstances are no longer the focus. The focus is now on potential, possibility, and future. Today the world needs more courageous souls that do more than just talk of hope, but live hope with action. The eyes that portray hunger for hope are the same across the world. It is a hunger that has existed since the beginning of time. I, for one, am committed to being a feeder of hope during my time on this planet. By the way, I have also learned that a generous giver of hope is, in turn, a bountiful receiver of hope. I am tired from the journey, but filled with a renewed passion to live as a role model of hope. Here's to a fresh batch of hope to you my friend. I encourage you to join me in being a feeder of hope.

7 Ways Parents Mislead Their Children without Even Knowing It

After raising 3 children, I found that being a parent is very tough. Having made numerous mistakes, I cannot say I am perfect. However, I have learned a few things.

I am sorely saddened by the state of childhood obesity. We address it with public service announcements or revamped school cafeteria menus, among other initiatives. Being a naturopathic doctor, I am always looking at the underlying causes of any issue. In the case of childhood obesity, I need not look further than the parents. I encourage you as a parent, or prospective parent, to take a long and honest look at each of the following examples of what is going on in our world today.

7 Ways Parents Mislead Their Children

1. Parents give their children candy because they want it and will not be quiet until they get it.
2. Parents stop by the nearest fast food restaurants because they do not have the time or desire to cook.
3. Once at the fast food restaurant, the parents ask the child what they want.
4. If a meal is cooked and the child does not like the selection, the parents will cook another meal just so the child will eat.
5. Parents discourage physical activity by 'plugging' their children in to all the newest electronic entertainment… just because every body else does it.
6. If a child is overweight, parents do not address it because they, themselves, are overweight or obese.
7. Parents remain naive by ignoring the health risks their children are facing by encouraging behavior that increases the likelihood for obesity.

I Limitless Strength

So, do those sound familiar? How many are synonymous with your own behavior? Do they seem overwhelming in nature?

I know this issue is difficult, so let's address it head on. First, take the initiative by *apologizing to your children* and owning your responsibility as a parent. After all, a parent's job is to nurture, lead, guide, provide, and protect. Following are ways to combat the 7 issues stated above.

7 Ways to Lead Your Children the Right Way

1. Candy is not a necessity for life. If does nothing to promote health, and it *not* a reward. It is actually a punishment.
2. Plan better and do not be too lazy to cook. You control the schedule. Your child's job is not to run things.
3. Select the food your kids *need*, not what the want. Protect them, please!
4. If the child doesn't eat, they will be hungry. Trust me, they will learn to eat what you cook.
5. Walk or exercise with your children. Limit the electronic time to 1 hour daily or less. The children will love and appreciate you so much for this later in life.
6. Be honest about your own weight or health condition. Do something about it. It is funny how people will say "you are too skinny" but few ever say "you are too fat."

7. Don't kill your children with neglect. Don't you really want them to be more healthy than you when they grow? If yes, then help them as opposed to serving them a plate full of setbacks.

Please be encouraged and inspired to take a stand now against childhood obesity. Do not let it affect your family any longer. Be a parent...be a leader! This, my friend, is who you were designed to be.

Reinventing Integrity

Integrity! What exactly does it mean to have integrity? And...where oh where has it gone? In a world of uncertainty and unpredictability, where can we look in regard to finding integrity? To answer these questions and more, we must first determine the meaning of integrity. According to Webster's Dictionary, integrity is:

1. firm adherence to a code of especially moral or artistic values: incorruptibility
2. an unimpaired condition: soundness
3. the quality or state of being complete or undivided: completeness

In this definition we see an overall theme of character, morality, and uprightness. Does this sound like a common

| Limitless Strength

theme today? To me, the answer is simple–WE HAVE FELL PREY IN SOCIETY TO A DETERIORATION OF INTEGRITY. I am not immune. Sadly, I must admit falling short in all areas during the course of my time on earth. However, it does not preclude me from beginning afresh each day with a renewed desire to live a life of integrity. Friend, neither should your own misgivings stop you from doing better each day.

We must REINVENT INTEGRITY into the fabric of our lives first THEN into the fabric of our society. So how do we spur the re-ignition of the integrity fire in our own lives? Here are some simple and practical keys that are certain to nurture integrity:

1. Guard your words! Choose the words you speak wisely and with great thought. Pause before you speak. Don't just spout off at the mouth without thinking. Many times we speak without regard to the truth. Think carefully before you answer questions. Is it the truth or not? SPEAK THE TRUTH, and let your YES be YES and your NO be NO. We try so hard to impress others; we weave stories that are greatly exaggerated. Make sure your words are like trusted gems that can be considered valuable and trustworthy.

2. Return calls! This is highly disrespectful to others when you do not return calls. It says loudly, "I don't have any value for you or your time." It further echoes, "I am

much more important than you and do not have time for you." I know these words sound strong, but that is exactly the interpretation from NOT RETURNING CALLS or messages. Email is much the same way. It is the theme of disrespect that must be halted. By returning calls and messages, you will build trust and show massive amounts of integrity in a world that is sorely in lack.

3. Arrive on time! DO NOT BE LATE! If you are late, you again are showing great disrespect for another's time. If you set an appointment, do it with thought and do not over-schedule where being late is likely. What this means is—GIVE YOURSELF PLENTY OF TIME TO BE ON TIME. I was taught that being 15 minutes early is being on time. If you are going to be late, at least call and let the person know. DO NOT THINK THAT BEING LATE IS OK. It never was and never will be! In a society where being late is expected, BE ON TIME. You will be greatly bless the other person by your promptness.

4. Do not overspend! Don't spend more than what you make and live within your means. This will be a great stress reliever for you and others around you. It will shape your integrity by learning to say NO because your bank account doesn't allow. A good rule of thumb is this—LIVE IN AGREEMENT WITH YOUR ASSETS. If you don't have the assets, don't

❦ | Limitless Strength

create debt. Overspending in trying to keep up with the Jones', has ruined the integrity of our society. Trust me; you will have MUCH more in the long run by learning to live within your budget day by day.

5. Say PLEASE and THANK YOU often! Showing gratitude is equivalent to having personal integrity. We are all so blessed that taking the blessing for granted is commonplace. We can do better. Simply by making requests with the inclusion of PLEASE and receiving blessing with words of THANKS, can add integrity to the very atmosphere. PLEASE and THANK YOU show tremendous respect and honor to the people in which you deal.

6. Own your failures! It is NOT SOMEONE ELSE'S FAULT, ALL THE TIME. This a big problem today. We live in a society of blame deflection. It is very healthy, but painful, to own your OWN FAILURES. If you make a mistake (and WE ALL WILL), just own it. If retribution is necessary, do it. If punishment is deserved, serve it. Always own it and offer heartfelt apologies. Saying, "I am sorry," can be a very freeing experience. Don't follow the apology with the word BUT. That negates the entire thing and minimizes the original offense. Follow the apology with a PERIOD! Owning your own failures is a critical key to the development of integrity.

Reinventing integrity is rebuilt one brick at a time. Integrity is not built overnight, especially when it has been damaged. In a society where integrity is collapsing, let's make a real commitment to rebuild it and reinvent it in our own lives. Put these described steps into practice one day at a time. Do not get ahead of yourself. Just take it ONE STEP AT A TIME. Over time, the foundation of integrity will be reinvented in your life and become a mighty fortress of exemplary legacy for a long time to come.

The Art of Uncommon Courtesy

During a recent visit to the post office, I saw a woman holding several packages in her arms as she approached the front entry doors. Without thinking, I quickly opened the door for her and said, "There you go ma'am." She looked me with a shocked and stated, "Why thank you young man. People just don't do those things anymore."

I went away from that experience thinking about the lady's response to what I thought was a common chivalrous gesture. However, the more I thought about it, I realized the lady may indeed be correct. Have we (as men) forgotten chivalry? Have we in effect 'killed it' by not making it the norm?

Listen, chivalry isn't dead unless YOU decide to kill it. Here are some simple, though apparently now uncommon, acts of chivalry that can be modeled and taught to children:

_❦_ | Limitless Strength

1. Open doors—whether someone has a load in their hands or not, it is still polite to open doors for ladies.

2. Return calls when you say you will—Be a person of honor. Call when you say you will, or you better have an important reason (that you can explain) why you did not.

3. Make a habit to say "yes ma'am, no ma'am, yes sir, no sir" to elders—This is so uncommon. Please utilize these words of respect often. They will carry you far.

4. Make sure your friends/spouse make it home OK—after you part ways with someone, make sure they make it home OK. It shows you are responsible and that you care.

5. Offer a coat if it's cold—don't be a blanket or coat hog. If someone with you is cold, lend your coat.

6. Get the car if it is raining—don't let someone get soaked. This is elementary, but unfortunately, some can be so selfish they totally ignore another's hard work on their hair and makeup. They went to a lot of trouble to look pretty for YOU.

7. Make your friends/spouse feel safe—Step in politely in an awkward situation. Show some courage and your protective side while still being polite and professional. You are trying to reduce conflict, not start it.

8. Don't be flaky or undependable—Be predictable. It is very important that people know what to expect.

9. Show interest in him/her—ask questions and LISTEN. Pay attention to the response and make sure your body language shows interest.
10. Show respect—Always value the other person. You will not agree with everyone about everything. Listen to others opinions, give your own if requested, and always show respect.

There you have it; 10 easy to follow acts of chivalry. Put these on your wall in your home or office. Utilize them, and I guarantee you will generate a constant flow of joy. Don't kill chivalry! Let's give it a fresh rebirth and start a chivalrous generation.

Who Else Wants More Time?

As we age, it seems as though time picks up speed. We go faster and faster and then wonder where time went. We pack our schedules and 'to do lists' so tight that we are literally begging for more time…and very upset that we don't have it. At the end of most days, we may find ourselves very restless and panicked because we were unable to complete all the day's tasks or obligations.

Do any of these (or most) statements match your current life circumstance? If they do, I have some surefire time-saving concepts to make your life a bit easier. Are you ready for more time? If so, incorporate the following:

8 Time-Saving Tricks to Make Your Life Easier

1. **Begin with the day ahead.** The way you begin your day is a great indicator of how you will finish. With that said, begin the day ahead. To accomplish this, set each clock in your house 15 minutes fast. Do not forget to include you cell phone, watch, and car clock. This will help you *not* be late.

2. **Set two alarms in the morning.** One alarm can be at bedside if you choose, but the second needs to be across the room. This will force you to get out of bed to shut it off.

3. **Have your coffee ready when you wake up.** If you are a morning coffee drinker, utilize a preset feature to have your coffee brewing at the time you awake. This will ensure the nice, hot 'wake up' drink will be waiting for you.

4. **Develop a prioritized to do list.** Make it routine to carry around a small notebook designed with all your daily 'to do' items. Put a big star by the highest priority items. Next to the star, rank the items in list of greatest priority by inserting a 1, 2, 3, etc. Your job is then to accomplish them in order. Do not get distracted. As things pop up throughout the day, just add them to the list and adjust priority if needed. When one is accomplished, mark it out where you actually see one less thing to do.

5. **Clear your mind at the end of the day.** At the end of each day, make sure you 'brain dump' all things to accomplish tomorrow in your notebook. Do not simply commit it to memory…make a new list. This simple task is aided by putting your small notebook in the bathroom, which is normally the last place we visit before bedtime.

6. **Practice the skill of saying NO.** Sometimes saying yes to others is saying no to yourself. We can over commit in this way and then we just have a bad attitude. Additionally, oftentimes we enable others in a negative way by not letting them figure it out for themselves. Remember, it is *not* your job to fix anybody. Bottom line…sometimes yes is in order but not *all* the time.

7. **Pick your clothes the night before.** That's right! Set out tomorrow's clothing tonight.

8. **End your day with 10 minutes of silence.** Spend at least 10 minutes of silent time in prayer, meditation, or just plain quiet each evening before bed. This will allow a much needed time of introspection and inner healing to occur. Oftentimes, this creates an amazing peace and is one of the best uses of time.

Begin utilizing these eight concepts today. It will make tomorrow easier and get you on the road to being back in charge of your life.

Heroes Wanted

Historically, heroes are memorialized because of incredible actions, lives, or legacy. Heroes give their lives for a cause, have immeasurable passion, and indescribable courage. They stand out from the crowd, they speak up when no one else will, and they step up to heights few have ever experienced. By those descriptors, a hero is a rare breed indeed.

Today, like no other time in history, WE are all in need of heroes. In an age of political correctness and fear of creating offense, few rise to the aforementioned levels. Is it because of fear, lack of passion, frustration? I am certain all of these, and more, become validated excuses. My friends, it is time to eliminate the excuse and stand up. We must not be fearful and not allow passions to be extinguished. Principles, morals, and ethics represent worthwhile heroic cause. Who will stand in the gap for the future, our children, and the legacy in which they represent? I hope and pray it is YOU.

As for me, my faith is important. I do not back down. At the same time, I will not cram it down someone else's throat. That action in itself can cause the taste to become bitter with irreversible damage. With that said, here are 3 key principles to rekindling the hero inside of YOU:

1. Let faith be your guide—this is done with actions, not words. Words are clanging gongs without corresponding actions. The best 'sermons' of faith I

have ever heard are the ones I have seen. Don't tell me what you are doing; show me what you are going to tell me. Your faith will begin to speak in your actions and become a guide to you and others.

2. Speak up in love–if you do not agree with something, speak up about it in love rather that condemnation. Condemnation will get you nowhere. Choose your words wisely and do not allow emotion to prompt regretted verbiage. Do not be afraid of creating offense. If love is your guide and offense occurs, love will know how to appropriately handle the other person/group. Remember, offense is often sign of internal conflict expressed outward, and it has little to do with you.

3. Moralistic and ethical behavior is important– morals are formed to keep us from harm. When we compromise morals and ethics, societal decay is certain. We are currently observing many signs of societal decay in this area. Our country was founded on God, faith, morals, and ethics. No matter what you or I think, we should not be deceived to believe otherwise. Crafty political savvy has steered us wrong. We, in the USA, are all blessed by this premise and order. Our founding fathers heroically stood up for the principles. Sacrifice was made, blood was shed, and God's blessing is clear. These principles are important and deserve protection.

The term 'hero' is not just for the few. It is for YOU and I. Friend, rekindle the courage, fight the good fight, speak in love, have a backbone, and do not back down on your principles. Let's all stand in the gap for our future. YOU will be honored, and the hero inside of you will appear and rise up.

3 Keys That Will Lead You to Greatness

Greatness…it's really what we all desire. In order to really have the opportunity to be *great*, we must first understand what it is. Greatness is defined as: the quality of being great, distinguished, or eminent. Some synonyms are eminence, distinction, illustriousness, repute, or high standing. That does indeed sound like a worthy goal. Even more appealing is the opportunity to leave a great legacy. With a basic working knowledge of greatness, one can now dive in to and embrace 3 keys to being great.

Key 1: Be fully committed.

You cannot be "wishy-washy" and become great. Commitment is important because it carries you past failure and into opportunity. When you fail at something, the tendency is to give up and try something else. That is the very epitome of "wishy-washy." If you are committed to something, you WILL NOT QUIT. Greatness does not soak in failure. Greatness seizes failure by the tail and turns it to opportunity to begin again. You can and should take lessons from failure, but rather than focus on the failure, focus on the lessons. Remain committed at all cost and you will see great dividends.

Key 2: Remain consistent.

Being consistent is about being predictable. People need to know what to expect when it comes to you. To lack consistency is to lack predictability. If other people have no idea what to expect from you, you may be known as "flighty." Further, if you are unpredictable to others, you are quite likely unpredictable to yourself. Being consistent is simplified by setting (and sticking to) a schedule. There is really very little chance of being consistent without setting a schedule. In the world in which we live, distractions are commonplace. Avoid distraction, set your schedule, be predictable and live consistently.

Key 3: Cultivate the right relationships.

With whom you frequent your time is critical. I cannot underestimate the importance of correct companionship. There are basically two types of persons in the world: eagles and vultures. Eagles soar above the storms. They fly higher and observe things from a larger, more panoramic view. Eagles do not make their home at the bottom. They make their home on top. They do not use others as stepping stools, and they do not let others hold them back. Vultures, on the other hand, hide

Limitless Strength

in the crags of rocks. They stay in the storms until the storms pass, all the while waiting on the next storm. The eat from the bottom and are very comfortable with ingesting seconds or others spoils. Be a companion of eagles rather than vultures. Invest your time with those who pull you higher instead of those who pull you down. By doing this habitually, you will find yourself soaring without assistance.

Allow these three keys to infiltrate not only your head, but your heart. These keys are critical and cannot be ignored or glossed over. 2 out of 3 is NOT good enough if you want to be great. Post these keys in a conspicuous place and daily make them your purpose. Greatness will soon follow. My friend, *you were created for greatness* and nothing less.

Life without Impossibility

How many times in life have we heard the statement, "You can't do that"? As for me, I have heard it plenty and many times it has been directed at me. Words are powerful, and words leave last scars. On the flip side, words can also leave lasting stars. There may indeed be things you CAN'T do, which can be for a variety of reasons. However, I want you to hear something else: "It is not what you CAN'T do the matters; it is what you CAN do that matters."

You must live with a CAN DO attitude to truly live life without impossibility. A 'CAN'T DO' attitude is the foundation of all failure.

213

Let's face it...limitations are real, but it doesn't mean the limitations create impossibility. Here are some keys to eliminating your own limits and living with possibility:

1. You must get control of you. You cannot lead someone to a place you have never been. Live it first. Embrace the experience, and practice what you preach. Understanding you are not perfect, DO NOT live an intentional hypocritical life.
2. Your change starts on the inside with what you put in your mind. Fill your mind and thoughts with CAN DO positivity. Evaluate–Is your life, your family a place where positivity reigns? If not, why not?
3. Inner change brings outer results. Real and genuine results gain attention and garner great influence. True and LASTING change does not begin on the outside. It does not come from a doctor, preacher, pill, or diet. It is the heart change that brings results.
4. Outer results fuels greater influence. You want to really impact the world? Show people authentic results. Folks want to see genuineness. What have you been through, and what roads have you traveled?

Incorporate these four keys in your life. Then, you may write your story without impossibility. Have you thought about the title of your life story? What are the chapters,

♥ | Limitless Strength

subplots, subtleties? Is it a mystery or inspiration? YOU hold the pen. YOU make it what you want.

You CAN DO it!

Nothing can stand in your way of a positive life filled with a path of conquered obstacles and limitless victories.

Extra Spiritual Wellness Nuggets

How Do We Understand Evil?

As I ponder the horrific incidents of violent activity in the world today, my emotions nearly spiral out of control. I want to understand, but I don't. I want to get mad, but at whom? After taking a break to be quiet and listen, I sense these words coming out:

The tears flow from deep inside. The cries of "WHY?" scream from the depths of our heart. We struggle to find explanation and rationalization to understand evil. We plead with the government to establish laws to prevent this evil from obtaining mechanisms to carry it out. We blame societal flaws, economic uncertainty, and overall desperation. In our attempt to 'understand,' we seek answers from outside of ourselves. The pursuit of this explanation has been a centuries-long pursuit that began with Cain killing his brother Abel. Why did that happen? What is the real reason? Was it simple jealousy or does it go much deeper?

In reality, there is NO outer explanation for evil. It is not the fault of guns, knives, bombs, advocacy groups, politicians, or law makers. Let us all take a hard look in the mirror. Let the reflection in the mirror pierce into our inner parts. What is really inside a man? Remember, nobody taught us how to lie, hold resentment, or become angry when we don't get our way. Evil is present in the very core of our inner being. It IS there whether we really want to admit it. It is planted and can grow. If it is not tended, it will grow out of control and consume.

As we observe a worldly trend of increasing heights of evil, we need not look farther for explanations and answers than square in the mirror. We MUST tend (and prune) the evil within by first admitting it IS there. By continuing to look outside, we ignore the inside and lose sight of the only thing we REALLY have control over—ourselves. By careful self-examination, the inside garden of evil can be observed, recognized, and managed.

The tears will continue to flow as evil WILL continue its presence. However, by recognizing the true source of evil, our efforts to find explanation and understanding may prove somewhat fruitful. In those efforts, we find that our inner eyes will become directed to the only source of peace, the only remedy for evil, and the only answer to our problem— God. Peace can only be found be seeking Him. Let us not forget that God, and God alone, created man, and provides eternal hope.

Is Our Faith a Private Matter?

This question has been a topic of conversation and point of contention for a number of years. Some stand on one side with great passion while others stand at any point in between. Let me take a few moments to expound on the question.

First, my country, the USA, was fundamentally founded on the principle of "In God We Trust." Notice the word "WE". That appears as a group as a WHOLE…meaning the founding fathers of this country adopted this motto as they represented the ENTIRE country. Further, "**In God We Trust**" was adopted as the official motto of the United States in 1956 as an alternative or replacement to the unofficial motto of E Pluribus Unum, adopted when the Great Seal of the United States was created and adopted in 1782.

"In God we trust" has appeared on most U.S. coins since 1864 and on paper currency since 1957.

Since our country placed its' trust in God publicly as the founder and provider of freedom, opportunity, and security, I wonder how faith becomes private? You see, faith and trust are tied together. You cannot have faith unless you have trust and vice versa. Obviously, the founders felt PUBLICLY confident in taking this stance. Notice the use of the word "God". It is a capital "G" rather than a small "g". This clearly brings us to the public presentation of the one and only GOD, who is the creator of the world and all mankind.

Sadly, we hear rumblings today about removing God from our money. So far, some have removed Him from our homes, jobs, and schools. What are the results? I do not have the time to write about ALL the detrimental effects. We have seen our country morally and ethically slide, people resort to unfathomable levels of evil, and some of the greatest tragedies in human history.

We talk of keeping our faith a private matter as to not offend anyone. It seems that our desire to do this has caused the offense to be self-inflicted. I would rather have someone stand against faith—YES even atheism—then stand for NOTHING. If you stand for nothing (as to not offend—or remaining 'private in the matter'); you can fall for anything. Haven't we fallen as a country far enough? Our fear of the public faith stance has made us, as a nation, our own worst enemy.

Additionally, I am bold enough to point out that Jesus, GOD'S SON (yes the same God in which WE place our trust), died a very public death on a cross. This is historically true, but also very important as it relates to our public stand on faith. He died for our sins (in which we are born into); he paid the price that we deserved to pay; he rose again from the dead so that WE could have life in Him. That life represents an eternity in the presence of GOD. The life, death, and resurrection of Jesus were PUBLIC.

Why should our faith be private? Only if we are afraid to take a stand and only if we are afraid to face truth. My faith is public. It is NOT private.

❦ | Limitless Strength

Friends, my country and my life was founded on public faith in GOD. Our blessings, opportunities, and hope we experience today are ALL authored by God. If he didn't create it and allow it, it would NOT happen. We can accomplish NOTHING without Him. We may try to say faith is a private matter. However, the more we act on that premise, the worst things become for us. I would not want to leave this earth without having a PUBLIC FAITH in which I boldly stand. We can make loads of money, have much success, experience the entire world has to offer, and attain high levels of fame, but when we leave this earth, we will take nothing. There are NO TRAILER HITCHES on the rear ends of hearses.

So friend…Is your faith private or public?

Pastors and the Big Squeeze

(a special message for pastors and church leaders)

As a minister who has had the privilege of getting to know a few hundred pastors, it is rare when I come across a pastor who is not tired, anxiety ridden, stressed, sick, exhausted, or burned out. The following statistics (according to the *New York Times*—Aug. 1, 2010) bear out very concerning numbers:

"Members of the clergy now suffer from obesity, hypertension and depression at rates higher than most Americans. In the last decade, their use of antidepressants has risen, while their life expectancy has fallen. Many would change jobs if they could."

- 13% of active pastors are divorced.
- Those in ministry are equally likely to have their marriage end in divorce as general church members.
- The clergy has the second highest divorce rate among all professions.
- 23% have been fired or pressured to resign at least once in their careers.
- 25% don't know where to turn when they have a family or personal conflict or issue.
- 25% of pastors' wives see their husband's work schedule as a source of conflict.
- 33% felt burned out within their first five years of ministry.
- 33% say that being in ministry is an outright hazard to their family.
- 40% of pastors and 47% of spouses are suffering from burnout, frantic schedules, and/or unrealistic expectations.
- 45% of pastors' wives say the greatest danger to them and their family is physical, emotional, mental, and spiritual burnout.
- 45% of pastors say that they've experienced depression or burnout to the extent that they needed to take a leave of absence from ministry.

| Limitless Strength

- 50% feel unable to meet the needs of the job.
- 52% of pastors say they and their spouses believe that being in pastoral ministry is hazardous to their family's well-being and health.
- 56% of pastors' wives say that they have no close friends.
- 57% would leave the pastorate if they had somewhere else to go or some other vocation they could do.
- 70% don't have any close friends.
- 75% report severe stress causing anguish, worry, bewilderment, anger, depression, fear, and alienation.
- 80% of pastors say they have insufficient time with their spouse.
- 80% believe that pastoral ministry affects their families negatively.
- 90% feel unqualified or poorly prepared for ministry.
- 90% work more than 50 hours a week.
- 94% feel under pressure to have a perfect family.
- 1,500 pastors leave their ministries each month due to burnout, conflict, or moral failure.
- Doctors, lawyers and clergy have the most problems with drug abuse, alcoholism and suicide.

Obviously, there is something here that is not being addressed. Let's be very real for a few minutes and define what I call the BIG SQUEEZE. Pastors serve in a 24 hour on-call capacity. As a former police officer, I can relate. However, I actually got time off. I encouraged my fellow officers, whom I frequently educate, to take time away, find friends outside of law enforcement, and generate non-law enforcement hobbies. But, what about pastors? They get no time away. Because of the very nature of the characteristic of compassion, some may feel the ability to say "no" is not possible. They can never detach. Their lives are centered on ministry, ministry, ministry!!! We try to say, "Well, there is a cost to really serve God in the ministry." Really? Does this mean losing your family, friends, mind, emotional well-being, and possibly your life? I think NOT. The "big squeeze" is a powerful pressure that can crush most pastors. It is the pressure to always say YES, to meet everyone's needs, to never take a day off, to always serve, to never allowing someone to simply minister to them.

If I had my way, I would mandate that EVERY pastor take at least one Sunday off a month (with his/her family) and NOT go to church. Take a vacation or just sleep in. Unless a life or death emergency arises, do not answer the cell phone. Stay away from the email. Don't drive by the church. Get away and devote time to YOU. YOU, pastor, are extremely valuable. How can a pastor feed others when they are starving? How can a pastor give from their well when their well has been long dry?

It is time to wake up and break free from the bondage of the "big squeeze." Obviously, for Satan to attack the pastors is a great tactical scheme. We must recognize this for attack and put our defenses in place. God certainly wants pastors to take

❦ | Limitless Strength

time away. Look at the example of Jesus. He actually walked off by himself at times. If He did it, why should a pastor feel guilty for doing it too? People in the congregation and flock can be extremely needy. They can drain a pastor dry and suck the very life out of them. It is time to get away, get built up, get strong, and return to deal with the "big squeeze." Much like the pressure of the earth "squeezes" rock, the pressure of being in the ministry can "squeeze" the pastor. This pressure in the earth can crush or it can force the formation of a valuable and unique diamond.

Pastors, take time for YOU! The "big squeeze" can be turned around for your good. Value God and value YOU!

Physical Stewardship

When I mention the idea of physical stewardship, some of you may be wondering, "What the heck is he talking about?" I will define this idea while working backward to forward. Let me begin with the idea of stewardship. Stewardship is taking care of (being a 'good steward' of) the thing(s) which you have been given (given charge over or responsibility for).

If you are fortunate enough to have children, you will need to be a good steward of them. You would do what you could to help them, heal them, encourage them, and prepare them for life. Your love for them may prompt you to say that you would give your life for them. If you have a spouse, you should feel the same way. Your spouse and your kids are gifts to you. If you have a great job (that you love) which pays you lots of money and offers you great benefits, you would protect it at all costs. You wouldn't think of just walking into your boss' office one day and saying, "Take this job and shove it." Notice I did say a job YOU LOVE.

You have probably been correctly told that life itself is a gift. Do not take it for granted. Count your blessings. Each day is a miracle. What about the idea of physical stewardship? Friend, you have been gifted only ONE body. It is the only one you have. You cannot get a replacement. Both you and I need to realize we are to be 'physical stewards' of the body we have been given. Care for your body by feeding it proper nutrition and activating your muscles through regular exercise. Yes, the concept of stewardship is easily understandable, and it applies to your physical person as well. I encourage you to apply this idea DAILY to your physical self. Let your life exhibit PHYSICAL STEWARDSHIP.